Behavioural Neurology of Antiepileptic Drugs

To F.M., *maestro di color che sanno.*

Behavioural Neurology of Antiepileptic Drugs

A Practical Guide

Andrea E. Cavanna

Michael Trimble Neuropsychiatry Research Group, Birmingham and Solihull Mental Health NHS Foundation Trust and University of Birmingham, UK

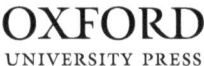

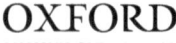
UNIVERSITY PRESS

Great Clarendon Street, Oxford, OX2 6DP,
United Kingdom

Oxford University Press is a department of the University of Oxford.
It furthers the University's objective of excellence in research, scholarship,
and education by publishing worldwide. Oxford is a registered trade mark of
Oxford University Press in the UK and in certain other countries

© Oxford University Press 2018

The moral rights of the author have been asserted

Frist Edition published in 2018

All rights reserved. No part of this publication may be reproduced, stored in
a retrieval system, or transmitted, in any form or by any means, without the
prior permission in writing of Oxford University Press, or as expressly permitted
by law, by licence or under terms agreed with the appropriate reprographics
rights organization. Enquiries concerning reproduction outside the scope of the
above should be sent to the Rights Department, Oxford University Press, at the
address above

You must not circulate this work in any other form
and you must impose this same condition on any acquirer

Published in the United States of America by Oxford University Press
198 Madison Avenue, New York, NY 10016, United States of America

British Library Cataloguing in Publication Data

Data available

Library of Congress Control Number: 2017959065

ISBN 978–0–19–879157–7

Oxford University Press makes no representation, express or implied, that the
drug dosages in this book are correct. Readers must therefore always check
the product information and clinical procedures with the most up-to-date
published product information and data sheets provided by the manufacturers
and the most recent codes of conduct and safety regulations. The authors and
the publishers do not accept responsibility or legal liability for any errors in the
text or for the misuse or misapplication of material in this work. Except where
otherwise stated, drug dosages and recommendations are for the non-pregnant
adult who is not breast-feeding

Links to third party websites are provided by Oxford in good faith and
for information only. Oxford disclaims any responsibility for the materials
contained in any third party website referenced in this work.

Contents

Introduction *vii*

1	Behavioural co-morbidities in epilepsy	1
2	Antiepileptic drugs and behaviour: mechanisms of action	7
3	Carbamazepine, oxcarbazepine, and eslicarbazepine	21
4	Clonazepam and clobazam	39
5	Ethosuximide	49
6	Gabapentin	55
7	Lamotrigine	61
8	Levetiracetam, piracetam, and brivaracetam	69
9	Phenobarbital and primidone	77
10	Phenytoin	85
11	Pregabalin	93
12	Tiagabine	101
13	Topiramate	107
14	Valproate	115
15	Vigabatrin	123
16	Zonisamide	129
17	Other antiepileptic drugs: rufinamide, lacosamide, perampanel	135
18	Comparative evidence and clinical scenarios	147

References *151*
Index *159*

Introduction

> The good physician is concerned not only with turbulent brain waves but with disturbed emotions
>
> *William G. Lennox and Charles H. Markham (1953)*

> The clinical interface between psychiatry and neurology is epilepsy; the pharmacological expression of this interface is antiepileptic drugs, as they are used to treat both epilepsy and psychiatric disorders. [...] Regrettably, both psychiatrists and neurologists are not well versed in the antiepileptic drugs literature that comes from each other's specialty.
>
> *Kenneth R. Kaufman (2011)*

Antiepileptic drugs are among the most commonly prescribed medications by both neurologists and psychiatrists, as they exert a number of effects that extend far beyond their anticonvulsant properties. There is growing evidence that each antiepileptic drug is characterized by a specific behavioural profile: for example, the mood stabilizing properties demonstrated by valproate, carbamazepine, and lamotrigine have been recognized as useful psychotropic effects, resulting in regulatory indications for treating patients with bipolar affective disorder. The *Behavioural Neurology of Antiepileptic Drugs* provides the first clinically oriented reference book on the use of antiepileptic drugs with a focus on their behavioural effects in both patients with epilepsy and patients with primary psychiatric conditions.

This book aims to be a pocket-sized guide to assist neurologists in the use of antiepileptic drugs when treating patients with epilepsy and associated behavioural problems (ictal anxiety, post-ictal psychosis, interictal dysphoric disorder, to cite but a few). Needless to say, psychiatrists treating patients with affective, anxiety, and psychotic disorders will also find this compendium on the behavioural aspects of antiepileptic drugs a useful tool for their clinical practice. The book is organized alphabetically by antiepileptic drug for easier information gathering, enabling physicians to use the text as a standalone reference in busy clinical settings, such as specialist epilepsy clinics or general psychiatry ward rounds.

Particular care has been taken in covering the breadth of medications used in modern epilepsy and psychiatry practice, including each drug's indications, contra-indications, side-effects, and important interactions. The underlying pharmacology is also presented to provide a quick refresher and background on the underlying mechanisms. Practical aspects related to prescribing and therapeutic drug monitoring are covered following the most up-to-date evidence-based guidance. However, it is important to note that most recommendations on clinical practice in the field of behavioural symptoms in epilepsy are empirical, as data based on methodologically sound research are often lacking. Each drug monograph closes with a section providing a visual overall rating in terms of antiepileptic indications, behavioural tolerability, interactions in polytherapy, and psychiatric use, again drawing on the existing evidence. A selected reference list is included to provide the reader with the primary sources for clinically relevant information presented in a concise way within each chapter. Coherence is maintained by the use of a universal template for each drug, with consistency in both required information and writing style.

It was felt that a new agile and up-to-date book was acutely needed to fill the gap between existing neuropharmacology textbooks (which focus mainly on the anticonvulsant effects of antiepileptic drugs) and, often out-of-date, monographs (which summarize antiepileptic drugs' psychiatric indications for the psychiatry audience). This book's practical approach and pocket size makes it a particularly useful resource for medical practitioners working with adult patients in the United Kingdom, although its unique cross-disciplinary features make it a valuable reference for the global audience.

Inevitably, while striving to achieve the best compromise between comprehensiveness and conciseness, important omissions and inaccuracies will have occurred, and this will not have escaped the attention of more learned readers. The alphabetical list of antiepileptic drugs is far from being exhaustive; voluntary omissions encompass, for example, drugs that are more rarely prescribed, drugs for paediatric use, and drugs with a restricted market because of specific warnings. These factors have provided the rationale for the exclusion of a number of pharmacological agents, including acetazolamide, felbamate, retigabine, stiripentol, and tetracosactide (adrenocorticotropic hormone or ACTH). Moreover, it is important to note that this book was written with a specific readership (i.e. behavioural neurologists) in mind; this explains why the text does not cover a number of important topics, such as emergency medications used for the treatment of status epilepticus, psychopharmacology, and behavioural therapy of psychiatric disorders in co-morbidity with epilepsy. Likewise, more invasive procedures, such as epilepsy surgery have not been included in a manual focusing on the behavioural aspects of antiepileptic drugs. These aspects of epilepsy care fall outside the remits of specialists in behavioural neurology. The relatively high prevalence of behavioural symptoms in patients with epilepsy is a serious and very complex problem, with important implications in terms of health-related quality of life. It has been suggested that one potential solution is for neurologists is to begin therapeutic interventions for uncomplicated behavioural symptoms, including non-refractory mood and anxiety disorders that are not co-morbid with suicidal risk, personality disorders, substance abuse, bipolar disorder, or psychotic disorder. The first important step in the behavioural neurologist's intervention is the optimization of antiepileptic treatment in patients with epilepsy and co-morbid behavioural symptoms. Hopefully, the borderlands between neuropharmacology and psychopharmacology chartered in this book will offer unique insights and precious resources to treating clinicians who prioritize health-related quality of life as a therapeutic outcome for their patients. It does not appear anachronistic to refer to Lennox and Markham's 1953 statement that the patient with epilepsy 'is not just a nerve-muscle preparation; he is a person' as a guiding principle for the medical science of the new millennium.

Birmingham (UK), February 2017

CHAPTER 1

Behavioural co-morbidities in epilepsy

The pharmacology and use of antiepileptic drugs (AEDs) sits on the clinical interface between neurology and psychiatry. The presence and clinical relevance of behavioural problems in patients with epilepsy has long been recognized (Fig. 1.1).

Behavioural problems reported by patients with epilepsy often have a worse impact on patients' health-related quality of life than the actual seizures. The treatment of patients with epilepsy is therefore not restricted to the achievement of seizure freedom, but must incorporate the management of psychiatric and cognitive co-morbidities. Epilepsy, behaviour, and cognition have a complex relationship, which has a direct bearing on their respective management and has to be factored into the selection AEDs. Different AEDs can, in turn, affect the clinical presentation of behavioural and cognitive symptoms in patients with epilepsy in both a positive and negative way. Behavioural symptoms in epilepsy have a multifactorial aetiology, with pharmacotherapy being only one of several risk factors encompassing neurobiological and psychosocial domains. It has been recommended that, in addition to identifying the main psychiatric co-morbidities in patients with epilepsy, behavioural neurologists initiate treatment interventions for mild affective disorders, anxiety disorders presenting as generalized anxiety disorder and panic attacks, and mild cognitive problems. Optimization of the pharmacological treatment of the seizure disorder is the first step in the therapeutic pathway and should be based on the following parameters:

- patient's demographic data and epilepsy data (seizure type, epileptic syndrome);
- behavioural and cognitive profiles of the AED, AED's interaction profile, and impact on reproductive functions;
- presence of co-morbid neurological disorders and medical conditions.

Every aspect of the patient's history and knowledge of the AED's properties (including pharmacokinetic and pharmacodynamics properties that may yield potential therapeutic and/or iatrogenic effects) should be considered in the formulation of a comprehensive and individualized treatment plan.

"Melancholics ordinarily become epileptics, and epileptics, melancholics: what determines the preference is the direction the malady takes [...] if it bears upon the body, epilepsy, if upon the intelligence, melancholy"
Hippocrates, 410 BC

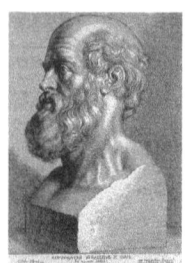

"He who is faithfully analysing many different cases of epilepsy is doing far more than studying epilepsy [...] A careful study of the varieties of epileptic fits is one way of analysing this kind of representation by the 'organ of mind'"
John Hughlings Jackson, 1888

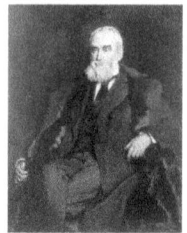

"Temporal lobe epilepsy is a probe for the study of the physiology of emotion, and opens up many possibilities for research"
Norman Geschwind, 1977

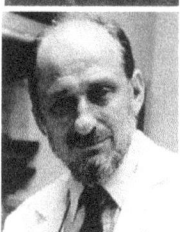

Fig. 1.1 Landmark quotes on the relationship between epilepsy and behaviour

Epidemiology and classification

Patients with epilepsy have a high prevalence of psychiatric co-morbidity compared with the general population and patients with other chronic medical conditions. Psychiatric co-morbidities of clinical significance are relatively frequent in the epilepsy population, affecting between 30 and 50% of patients. Affective and anxiety disorders are the most frequent psychiatric co-morbidities in patients with epilepsy, with lifetime prevalence rates of up to 35%. Although psychotic disorders are reported less frequently, their prevalence rates are higher than in the general population (7–10% versus 0.4–1% in the general population). The presence of co-morbid non-epileptic attack disorder (sometimes referred to as 'psychogenic non-epileptic attacks') can result in significant diagnostic challenges, whereas the association between temporal lobe epilepsy and specific personality traits (temporal lobe epilepsy personality disorder or 'Gastaut–Geschwind syndrome') is still controversial.

Psychiatric disorders reported by patients with epilepsy are often classified according to the temporal relationship with seizures—inter-ictal, peri-ictal (pre-ictal, ictal, post-ictal), and para-ictal symptomatology. The multifactorial aetiology of behavioural problems in epilepsy includes iatrogenic psychiatric conditions that are actually triggered by pharmacological interventions (behavioural profiles of AEDs). In general, the psychotropic effects of AEDs are thought to result from multiple factors related to the individual drug's mechanism(s) of action, the underlying neurological condition (especially if there is involvement of the limbic system), and the patient's clinical presentation and history. The early recognition and initial evaluation of behavioural symptoms in patients with epilepsy is crucial to formulate a comprehensive treatment plan that can target each condition.

Inter-ictal disorders

Affective and anxiety disorders

Most co-morbid inter-ictal affective and anxiety disorders do not present with specific distinguishing features that separate them from primary psychiatric conditions seen in the community. These co-morbid psychiatric disorders should therefore be classified using conventional diagnostic criteria [e.g. Diagnostic and Statistical Manual for Mental Disorders (DSM)]. However it should be noted that patients with epilepsy are more likely to develop specific types of phobias, such as fear of seizures, agoraphobia, and social phobia, as a result of recurrent seizures. Unlike primary psychiatric disorders, co-morbid phobias often revolve around epilepsy, and the fear of the situation and subsequent avoidance are linked to the fear of having a seizure, and its possible consequences. Likewise, specific intermittent affective and somatoform symptoms are frequently reported by patients with chronic epilepsy; these include irritability, depressive moods, anergia, insomnia, atypical pains, anxiety, phobic fears, and euphoric moods. These symptoms tend to follow a fluctuating clinical course and tend to last from a few hours to 2–3 days (sometimes longer). The presence of at least three intermittent dysphoric symptoms causing impairment indicates a diagnosis of inter-ictal dysphoric disorder. Inter-ictal dysphoric disorder is a homogenous construct that can be diagnosed in a relevant proportion of patients with epilepsy, possibly occurring in other central nervous system disorders, such as migraine.

Self-report screening instruments are useful psychometric tools to assist behavioural neurologists in the assessment of affective and anxiety disorders in patients with epilepsy. The Neurologic Depressive Disorder Inventory in Epilepsy (NDDI-E) is a six-item scale with a total score range of 6–24, where a score above 15 is suggestive of a diagnosis of depression. The Patient Health Questionnaire-Generalized Anxiety Disorder-7 is a seven-item scale with a total score range of 0–21, where a score above 10 suggests the diagnosis of generalized anxiety disorder. Both instruments are user-friendly and can be completed by patients in less than 5 minutes at each neurological consultation.

Psychosis

Chronic schizophrenia in patients with epilepsy can present with specific clinical features, which justify the definition of 'schizophrenia-like psychosis of epilepsy'. This condition resembles paranoid psychosis and is characterized by strong affective components, but not necessarily affective flattening. Behavioural symptoms may include command hallucinations, third-person auditory hallucinations, and other first-rank symptoms. Negative symptoms are rarely reported by patients with epilepsy and delusions are often characterized by a preoccupation with religious themes. There is a consensus that schizophrenia-like psychosis of epilepsy is characterized by lesser severity and better response to therapy than primary schizophrenia. Moreover, delusions and hallucinations in patients with epilepsy have been described as 'more empathizable', because 'the patient remains in our world'. Overall, there is a better premorbid function and rare deterioration of the patient's personality compared with other forms of schizophrenic psychosis.

Peri-ictal disorders

Peri-ictal disorders encompass behavioural symptoms that are temporally related to the actual seizures, and are classified as pre-ictal, ictal, and post-ictal. Although these symptoms have been recognized since the 19th century, they often go unrecognized.

Pre-ictal disorders

Pre-ictal psychiatric symptoms can herald a seizure and typically present as dysphoric mood (changes in mood with symptoms of anxiety and irritability, short attention span, and impulsive behaviour). These symptoms can precede a seizure by a period ranging from several hours to up to 3 days; symptom severity worsens during the 24 hours prior to the seizure and remit post-ictally, although persistence for a few days after the seizure has been reported.

Ictal disorders

Ictal psychiatric symptoms are the direct clinical expression of seizure activity. They are usually classified as features of the seizures themselves—experiential auras of simple partial seizures encompass symptoms like anxiety and panic, hallucinations, and abnormal thoughts. Ictal fear or panic is the most frequently reported symptom, comprising 60% of ictal psychiatric symptoms, followed by ictal depression. Ictal fear can be misdiagnosed as panic attack disorder. There is a possible link between ictal psychiatric symptoms and temporal lobe seizures. Non-convulsive status can also present with prolonged behavioural changes and catatonic features.

Post-ictal disorders

Post-ictal psychiatric symptoms typically present after a symptom-free period ranging from several hours to up to 7 days (usually after 24–48 hours—the 'lucid interval') after a seizure (clusters of seizures, more rarely single seizures) and are relatively frequently reported by patients with treatment-refractory focal epilepsy. The symptom-free period between the seizure and the onset of psychiatric symptoms can lead to their misdiagnosis as inter-ictal phenomena. Post-ictal psychotic episodes can last from a few days to several weeks, but usually subside spontaneously after 1–2 weeks. Post-ictal psychosis is typically by patients with a seizure disorder lasting for more than 10 years and is often preceded by secondarily generalized tonic-clonic seizures. Post-ictal psychosis characteristically presents with affect-laden psychotic symptomatology, often with paranoid delusions with religious themes; affective features, as well as visual and auditory hallucinations, may also be present. Confusion and amnesia have occasionally ben reported in association with the behavioural symptoms. Other post-ictal psychiatric symptoms include anxiety, depression, and neurovegetative symptoms. These symptoms can last for 24 hours or more, and can overlap with other psychiatric symptoms. Of note, only post-ictal psychosis has been found to respond to pharmacological interventions, whereas symptoms of depression, anxiety, irritability, and impulsivity have proven refractory to treatment interventions. Complete remission of post-ictal psychiatric symptoms can only be achieved with full remission of the seizure disorder.

Para-ictal disorders

Para-ictal behavioural symptoms are a rare type of psychiatric disorders in patients with epilepsy. Of considerable clinical relevance is the phenomenon of 'forced normalization' or 'alternative psychosis'—the development of acute psychotic (and sometimes affective) symptomatology following seizure remission in patients with treatment-resistant epilepsy. Remission of the behavioural symptoms occurs upon the recurrence of epileptic seizures. Therefore, patients alternate between periods of clinically manifest seizures and normal behaviour, and periods of seizure freedom accompanied by behavioural symptoms, which are often accompanied by paradoxical normalization of the EEG. Forced normalization has been reported in association with the use of several AEDs, including ethosuximide, clobazam, vigabatrin. Although the phenomenon of forced normalization presenting in the form of a pure psychotic episode is relatively rare and has been estimated to occur in approximately 1% of patient with treatment-refractory epilepsy; its presentation as a depressive episode is believed to be more frequent. Moreover, forced normalization is often unrecognized, as confident diagnosis requires long-term follow-up of patients.

CHAPTER 2

Antiepileptic drugs and behaviour: mechanisms of action

Antiepileptic drugs (AEDs) suppress epileptic seizures through a variety of mechanisms of action and molecular targets involved in the regulation of neuronal excitability. The main pharmacological actions include modulation of ion (mainly sodium and calcium) conductance through voltage-gated channels located within the neuronal membrane, as well as facilitation of inhibitory (GABAergic) neurotransmission and inhibition of excitatory (glutamatergic) neurotransmission (Table 2.1). Of note, converging evidence indicates that these neurobiological mechanisms and targets are also implicated in the regulation of behaviour. This may explain why each AED is associated with a specific psychotropic profile.

The story of the modern pharmacological treatment of epilepsy began in 1857, when Sir Charles Locock, obstetrician to Queen Victoria, reported in *The Lancet* on his use of potassium bromide in 15 young women with 'hysterical epilepsy connected with the menstrual period' (possibly catamenial epilepsy). Interestingly, potassium bromide, the first AED in clinical use was associated with a constellation of behaviourally adverse effects; 'bromism', described as somnolence, psychosis, and delirium, has been extensively documented. Over time, the development of AEDs has been characterized by steep accelerations in drug development, which is unparalleled by other neuropsychiatric disorders, especially after the impressive expansion in licensed drugs over the last couple of decades. AEDs can be grouped into three categories, based on their chronology (Fig. 2.1). Phenobarbital, phenytoin, primidone, ethosuximide, carbamazepine, and valproate, together with the benzodiazepines with anticonvulsant activity clonazepam and clobazam, belong to first-generation AEDs (pre-1980s). The modern era focused on the systematic screening of many thousands of compounds against rodent seizure models and resulted in the global licensing, in chronological order, of vigabatrin, lamotrigine, gabapentin, topiramate, tiagabine, oxcarbazepine, levetiracetam, pregabalin, and zonisamide (second-generation AEDs). Piracetam is a pyrrolidone-derivative structurally related to levetiracetam, which is mainly used as a nootropic agent and has anticonvulsant properties with clinical applications limited to cortical myoclonus. Finally, AEDs marketed during the last few years (i.e. carbamazepine-related eslicarbazepine, levetiracetam analogue brivaracetam, rufinamide, lacosamide, perampanel, and others as they became available) are often referred to as third-generation AEDs. In addition to

Table 2.1 Summary of the main mechanisms of action of antiepileptic drugs (AEDs)

AEDs	Voltage–gated Na$^+$ channel blockade	Voltage–gated Ca^{++} channel blockade	Enhancement of GABA transmission	Inhibition of glutamate transmission	SV2A binding
Phenobarbital	–	?	+	+	–
Phenytoin	+	?	?	?	–
Primidone	–	?	+	+	–
Ethosuximide	–	+	–	–	–
Carbamazepine	+	?	?	+	–
Valproate	+	+	+	?	–
Clonazepam	–	–	+	–	–
Piracetam	–	?	–	+	+
Clobazam	–	–	+	–	–
Vigabatrin	–	–	+	–	–
Lamotrigine	+	+	?	+	–
Gabapentin	–	+	?	–	–
Topiramate	+	+	+	+	–
Tiagabine	–	–	+	–	–
Oxcarbazepine	+	+	?	+	–
Levetiracetam	–	+	?	?	+

Pregabalin	−	+	−	−
Zonisamide	+	+	?	−
Rufinamide	+	−	?	−
Lacosamide	+	−	−	−
Eslicarbazepine	+	−	+	−
Perampanel	−	−	−	−
Brivaracetam	−	−	−	+

+ = mechanism present; ? = mechanism possibly present; − = mechanism absent.

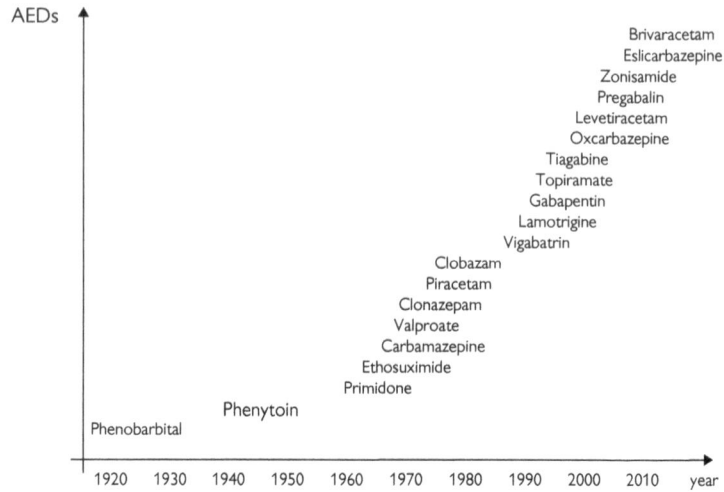

Fig. 2.1 Chronology of the clinical use of antiepileptic drugs (AEDs)

first- and second-generation AEDs currently used to treat adults with epilepsy, third-generation AED, which have demonstrated potential to become part of routine clinical practice, are covered in this book.

Phenobarbital

The pharmacological age of AED therapy began with the serendipitous discovery of the anticonvulsant properties of phenobarbital by young resident psychiatrist Alfred Hauptmann in 1912. Previously used for its hypnotic properties, phenobarbital is still the most widely prescribed AED in the developing world, partly because of its modest cost. Phenobarbital has an oral bioavailability of about 90%. Peak plasma concentrations are reached 8–12 hours after oral administration. Phenobarbital is one of the longest-acting barbiturates available, as it has a half-life of 50–120 hours and has very low protein binding (20–45%). Phenobarbital is mainly metabolized by the liver, through hydroxylation and glucuronidation, and induces many isozymes of the cytochrome P450 system. Phenobarbital is excreted primarily by the kidneys.

Through its action on GABA receptors, phenobarbital promotes GABA binding and increases the influx of chloride ions, thereby decreasing neuronal excitability. Direct blockade of excitatory glutamate signalling (presumably mediated by depression of voltage-dependent calcium channels) is also believed to contribute to the anticonvulsant and hypnotic effects observed with barbiturates. Phenobarbital features in the World Health Organization's List of Essential Medicines.

Phenytoin

Phenytoin was originally synthesized in 1908 by the German chemist Heinrich Biltz. In an effort to develop a less sedative AED than phenobarbital using the first electroencephalophic laboratory for the routine study of brain waves, Tracy Putnam and his young assistant Houston Merritt at the Boston City Hospital discovered the anticonvulsant properties of phenytoin in the 1930s. The absorption rate of phenytoin is dose-dependent and the time to reach steady-state is often longer than 2 weeks. The pharmacokinetic profile of phenytoin is characterized by mixed-order elimination kinetics at therapeutic concentrations. Phenytoin undergoes hepatic metabolism, but metabolic capacity can be saturated at therapeutic concentrations; below the saturation point, phenytoin is eliminated in a linear, first-order process, whereas above the saturation point, elimination is much slower and occurs via a zero-order process. Since elimination becomes saturated, a small increase in dose may lead to a large increase in phenytoin concentration. Because of the saturable metabolism, it would be inaccurate to report a fixed value for phenytoin half-life although, for most patients, a half-life of 20–60 hours may be found at therapeutic levels. The main mechanism of anticonvulsant action of phenytoin is mediated by inhibition of voltage-dependent sodium channels. Blockade of sustained high-frequency repetitive firing of action potentials is accomplished by reducing the amplitude of sodium-dependent action potentials through enhancing steady-state inactivation. Other mechanisms of action have been postulated, including inhibition of calcium influx across the cell membrane through voltage-gated calcium channels (especially when phenytoin is administered at higher doses). The primary site of action appears to be the motor cortex, where phenytoin inhibits the spreading of seizure activity. Overall, phenytoin exerts its anticonvulsant effects with less central nervous system sedation than does phenobarbital. Phenytoin features in the World Health Organization's List of Essential Medicines.

Primidone

Primidone is an AED of the barbiturate class. It is a structural analogue of phenobarbital, which is its main active metabolite. In Europe in the early 1960s it was not uncommon to prescribe primidone and phenobarbital in combination, often with a stimulant. Absorption of primidone is rapid but variable, and peak serum concentrations are reached within 3–4 hours. Primidone is bound only minimally to plasma proteins and its plasma half-life is 10–12 hours. Primidone is among the most potent hepatic enzyme-inducing drugs in existence; this enzyme induction occurs at therapeutic doses. The rate of metabolism of primidone into phenobarbital appears to be inversely related to age, with higher rates in older patients. The percentage of primidone converted to phenobarbital has been estimated to be 15% in humans. The exact mechanism of primidone's anticonvulsant action is still unknown. The main antiepileptic action of primidone is due to the major metabolite, phenobarbital, and it is possible that primidone itself and/or a second active metabolite, namely phenylethylmalonamide, contribute to its anticonvulsant properties.

Ethosuximide

Ethosuximide, developed after troxidone (an established treatment for patients with 'petit mal' during the 1940s), was introduced into practice in the late 1950s. Ethosuximide is completely and rapidly absorbed from the gastrointestinal tract, with peak serum levels occurring 1–7 hours after a single oral dose. Ethosuximide is not significantly bound to plasma proteins (less than 5–10%) and therefore the drug is present in saliva and cerebrospinal fluid in concentrations that approximate to plasma concentrations. The pharmacokinetic profile of ethosuximide is characterized by linear kinetics and this AED is extensively metabolized in the liver (cytochrome CYP3A4) to at least three plasma metabolites. Between 12 and 20% of the drug is excreted unchanged in the urine. The elimination half-life of ethosuximide is relatively long (40–60 hours in adults). The primary antiepileptic mechanism of action of ethosuximide is the blockade of conduction in low-voltage activated T-type calcium channels. Activation of the T-type calcium channels causes low-threshold calcium spikes in thalamic relay neurons, which are believed to play a role in the spike-and-wave pattern observed during absence seizures. Ethosuximide features in the World Health Organization's List of Essential Medicines.

Carbamazepine

Carbamazepine was synthesized in 1953 by chemist Walter Schindler at Geigy (now part of Novartis) in Basel, Switzerland, as a possible competitor for the recently introduced antipsychotic chlorpromazine. Carbamazepine is relatively slowly, but adequately absorbed after oral administration. The peak serum concentration of carbamazepine occurs at 4–5 hours and protein binding is approximately 75%. Its plasma half-life is about 30 hours (range 25–65 hours) when it is given as single dose. However, since carbamazepine is a strong inducer of hepatic enzymes, its plasma half-life shortens to about 15 hours (range 12–17 hours) when it is given repeatedly and induces its own metabolism. Over 90% of carbamazepine undergoes hepatic metabolism; its active metabolite is carbamazepine 10,11-epoxide. The multiple mechanisms of action of carbamazepine (and its derivatives oxcarbazepine and eslicarbazepine) are relatively well understood. Carbamazepine primarily acts as a blocker of use- and voltage-dependent sodium channels. Its possible role as a GABA receptor agonist may contribute to its efficacy in neuropathic pain and bipolar disorder. Carbamazepine's actions on voltage-gated calcium channels, as well as monoamine, acetylcholine, and glutamate receptors (NMDA subtype) have also been described. Moreover, laboratory research has shown that carbamazepine can act as a serotonin-releasing agent. Carbamazepine features in the World Health Organization's List of Essential Medicines, both as anticonvulsant, and as medicine used for mental and behavioural disorders.

Valproate

Valproic acid was first synthesized in 1882 by Beverly Burton as an analogue of valeric acid, found naturally in valerian. The antiepileptic properties of valproate were serendipitously recognized in 1963 by Pierre Eymard, while working as a research student at the University of Lyon. While using valproate as a vehicle for a number of other compounds that were being screened for antiseizure activity, he found that it prevented pentylenetetrazol-induced convulsions in laboratory rats. Valproate is absorbed rapidly and completely. Peak plasma concentrations after oral administration are usually reached within 1–5 hours. Valproate is mostly bound to plasma proteins (70–95%), and has a half-life of 7–20 hours. Valproate has complex pharmacokinetics, and is extensively metabolized in the liver, through oxidative and conjugation mechanisms, to biologically inactive metabolites. The clearance of valproate follows linear kinetics at most dosage ranges, but is increased at high doses, due to the higher free fraction of valproate. Although the mechanisms of action of valproate are not fully understood, its anticonvulsant effects have been mainly attributed to its inhibitory actions on calcium (low-threshold T-type channels) and potassium conductance, as well as blockade of voltage-dependent sodium channels and glutaminergic activity. It is believed that valproate increases brain concentrations of GABA through multiple pathways: the GABAergic effect is believed to contribute towards both its anticonvulsant and anti-manic properties. Valproate features in the World Health Organization's List of Essential Medicines both as anticonvulsant, and as medicine used for mental and behavioural disorders.

Clonazepam

The value of the benzodiazepines for the treatment of epilepsy was rapidly recognized following their synthesis and development by Leo Sternbach at Swiss pharmaceutical company Roche, in the 1960s. Clonazepam is a 1,4 benzodiazepine derivative and a chlorinated derivative of nitrazepam, a chloro-nitro benzodiazepine. This drug is extensively metabolized in the liver by cytochrome P450 enzymes into pharmacologically inactive metabolites, and has an elimination half-life of 19–50 hours (it is effective for 6–12 hours in adults). Clonazepam is largely (85%) bound to plasma proteins and passes through the blood–brain barrier easily, with blood and brain levels corresponding equally with each other. Clonazepam acts by binding to the benzodiazepine site of the GABA receptors, which enhances the effects of GABA binding on neurons by increasing GABA affinity for the GABA receptors. Binding of GABA to the site opens the chloride channel, resulting in an increased influx of chloride ions into the neurons and, therefore, in a hyperpolarization of the cell membrane, which prevents neuronal firing.

Piracetam

Piracetam was developed in 1967 by the research laboratory of UCB-Pharma in Belgium and marketed as a 'memory-enhancing drug' before its antimyoclonic effect was noted. Piracetam has an oral bioavailability of 100%, with a time to peak levels of 30–40 minutes. This drug is not bound to plasma proteins, does not undergo metabolism, and is completely excreted by the kidneys, with an elimination half-life of 5–6 hours. The modes of action of piracetam and most of its derivatives have not been fully elucidated. Piracetam weakly binds to the receptor of a synaptic vesicle protein known as SV2A, which is thought to be involved in synaptic vesicle exocytosis and presynaptic neurotransmitter release; this may be its main mechanism of action. Differential effects on subtypes of glutamate receptors, but not GABAergic action, have also been implicated. A further possible mechanism of piracetam is the facilitation of calcium influx into neuronal cells.

Clobazam

Clobazam is a 1,5 benzodiazepine derivative, and is probably the most widely used oral benzodiazepine for the treatment of epilepsies. Over 80% of the dose of clobazam is rapidly absorbed (peak serum concentrations reached within 1–4 hours) and its distribution volume increases with age. Clobazam is mostly (85%) protein bound, and is eliminated mainly by demethylation and hydroxylation pathways as part as hepatic metabolism. Its elimination half-life is in the order of 10–15 hours (longer in the elderly). The chronic effectiveness of clobazam may be predominantly due to its active metabolite, N-desmethylclobazam (norclobazam), which works by enhancing GABA-activated chloride currents at GABA-A receptor-coupled chloride channels. The modulation of GABA function in the brain by the benzodiazepine receptor leads to enhanced GABAergic inhibition of neurotransmission, similarly to clonazepam's action.

Vigabatrin

Vigabatrin, a close structural analogue of GABA, was marketed at the end of the 1980s as the prime example of a 'designer drug' engineered to produce a specific and rational mechanism of action, opening a new and fruitful chapter in epilepsy pharmacotherapy. After initial reports on vigabatrin's usefulness in the treatment of partial-onset seizures, the concerns about visual field defects resulted in a sharp decline in the use of this drug, saved only by the discovery of its value in infantile spasms. Vigabatrin has simple pharmacokinetics—absorption is rapid, with a peak concentration reached within 2 hours, and oral bioavailability is 60–70%, with no appreciable protein binding in plasma. The plasma half-life is 6–8 hours. Vigabatrin is distributed widely (volume of distribution 0.8 L/kg) and is only minimally metabolized in humans; elimination is primarily by renal excretion. Vigabatrin has a different mode of action from other AEDs: it binds irreversibly to GABA transaminase, the enzyme responsible for the metabolism of GABA within the synaptic cleft, resulting in its non-competitive inhibition.

Lamotrigine

During the 1960s, initial observations that patients with epilepsy treated with AEDs had diminished levels of folic acid led to the erroneous assumption that the antiepileptic effects of phenytoin and phenobarbital could be mediated through their antifolate properties. Lamotrigine, a triazine compound chemically unrelated to any other AED, was therefore developed as an antifolate drug. Although it is not characterized by a marked antifolate action, and there is no correlation between an anti-folate action and antiepileptic effects, lamotrigine was found to have a pronounced antiepileptic effect and was first introduced for the adjunctive treatment of focal seizures in the United Kingdom in 1991. Lamotrigine is rapidly absorbed orally, with a bioavailability approaching 100% and time to peak concentration within 1–3 hours after dosing. Protein binding is approximately 55% and less than 10% of the drug is excreted unchanged in the urine. Lamotrigine is metabolized in the liver via glucuronidation, without prior involvement of the CYP family of enzymes or generation of active metabolites. Elimination half-life is about 30 hours in monotherapy, 15 hours in polytherapy with glucuronidation inducers, 60 hours in polytherapy with valproate, and 25 hours in polytherapy with glucuronidation inducers and valproate. The mechanisms of action of lamotrigine include blockage of voltage-dependent sodium channel conductance (possibly associated with lamotrigine's antiglutamate and antiaspartate actions), modulation of voltage-dependent calcium conductance at N-type calcium channels and potassium conductance, and possible action on kynurenic acid, which may modulate the glycine binding site on the NMDA receptor.

Gabapentin

Although gabapentin was initially developed as a GABA analogue, it was later discovered that its antiepileptic effects are due to an entirely different mechanism— to its binding to the alpha2 delta1 subunit of voltage-activated calcium channels, which appears to be responsible for other beneficial effects on neuropathic pain and anxiety. There is some evidence that gabapentin might also increase GABA synthesis in humans. The bioavailability of gabapentin is only about 60% at lower doses and 35% or less at higher doses, as its gastrointestinal transporter is saturable (absorption varies considerably between individuals). Peak serum levels are achieved within 2–4 hours of oral dosing. Gabapentin is negligibly bound to plasma proteins and is eliminated entirely by renal excretion in an unchanged form, without hepatic metabolism, with an elimination half-life of 5–9 hours.

Topiramate

Topiramate is a monosaccharide derived from fructose, which was initially developed as an antidiabetic drug (it has only weak action in this regard) and was then found to have antiepileptic action after routine screening. Topiramate is quickly absorbed after oral use and achieves peak serum concentrations after 2 hours (range 1–4 hours). Protein binding is 15% (range 10–40%) and topiramate is mostly (70%) excreted in the urine unchanged, whereas the remainder is extensively metabolized by hydroxylation, hydrolysis, and glucuronidation. Six metabolites have been identified in humans, none of which constitutes more than 5% of the administered dose. Mean half-life is 21 hours (range 19–25 hours). Preclinical studies designed to elucidate the mechanisms of action of topiramate have identified a broad spectrum of pharmacological properties: blockade of voltage-dependent sodium channels, potentiation of GABA-mediated neurotransmission (by increasing the frequency at which GABA activates GABA-A receptors), inhibition of glutamate receptors (by antagonizing the ability of kainate to activate the kainate/AMPA subtype), negative modulatory effect on L-type calcium channels, and inhibition of carbonic anhydrase isoenzymes, plus effects on the phosphorylation state of membrane proteins.

Tiagabine

Tiagabine, the first of a series of 'GABA-wave' drugs to be introduced into clinical practice, was first marketed in the United Kingdom in 1998. Tiagabine is rapidly absorbed with excellent bioavailability. Unlike many of the other newer AEDs, tiagabine is highly bound to proteins (96%). Tiagabine is extensively metabolized by the hepatic cytochrome P450 isoenzyme CYP3A4, with less than 1% of the absorbed parent drug excreted unchanged. The serum half-life is 4–13 hours. Elimination is both renal and faecal. Tiagabine inhibits neuronal and glial reuptake of GABA by binding to recognition sites associated with the GABA uptake carrier. By blocking GABA reuptake into presynaptic neurons, tiagabine allows more GABA to be available for receptor binding on postsynaptic cells. However, despite considerable interest in tiagabine as a treatment of partial-onset seizures with a well understood and specific antiepileptic mode of action, it has been very little used in practice because of limited efficacy.

Oxcarbazepine

Oxcarbazepine is a keto-derivative of carbamazepine, in which an extra oxygen atom is added on the dibenzazepine ring. This difference avoids the epoxidation stage of metabolism, thereby reducing the risk of interactions, as well as bone marrow suppression and hepatic dysfunction. Oxcarbazepine is characterized by high bioavailability after oral administration. Upon absorption, oxcarbazepine is largely metabolized to its pharmacologically active 10-monohydroxy metabolite licarbazepine, which reaches peak serum concentration within 4–8 hours and has a protein binding of 40%. The half-life of oxcarbazepine is about 2 hours, whereas licarbazepine, which is the main responsible for the antiepileptic activity, has a half-life of 9 hours. Oxcarbazepine and licarbazepine exert their action by blocking voltage-sensitive sodium channels, thus leading to stabilization of hyperexcited neural membranes, suppression of repetitive neuronal firing, and decreased propagation of action potentials. Moreover, the anticonvulsant effects of these compounds could be attributed to enhancement of potassium conductance and modulation of high-voltage activated calcium channels, as well as possible modulation of glutamatergic neurotransmission (NMDA receptors).

Levetiracetam

Levetiracetam is one of a large family of pyrrolidone drugs and has a close structural similarity to piracetam. Early studies in other indications had used the racemic mixture, etiracetam. Levetiracetam is the L-enantiomer of etiracetam (the R-enantiomer being an inactive substance in models of epilepsy) and was marketed at the turn at the millennium under the trade name of Keppra® (UCB, Brussels, Belgium), after the Egyptian sun god. Levetiracetam is rapidly absorbed after oral administration, reaching its peak concentration at about 1 hour (range 0.5–2 hours) after ingestion. Its oral bioavailability approaches 100% and there is virtually no protein binding. In monotherapy, levetiracetam is largely (66%) excreted unchanged; most of the remainder (34%) is metabolized to a carboxylic acidic metabolite, which is inactive, and its metabolism does not involve the enzymes of the cytochrome P450 system. The half-life of levetiracetam in healthy people ranges between 5 and 8 hours. There is no autoinduction and the kinetics of levetiracetam is linear in clinical dose ranges. The mode of action of levetiracetam was initially unclear, but in 2004 a novel binding site (shared only by other pyrrolidone drugs, including piracetam) was identified—a synaptic vesicle protein known as SV2A, which is thought to be involved in synaptic vesicle exocytosis and presynaptic neurotransmitter release. Moreover, a subtype of N-type calcium channels appears to be sensitive to levetiracetam.

Pregabalin

Pregabalin was discovered in 1989 by the medicinal chemist Richard Silverman working at Northwestern University in Chicago. Pregabalin is rapidly absorbed, with peak plasma concentrations occurring within 1 hour (oral bioavailability is estimated to be at least 90%). There is no protein binding and the half-life is about 6 hours. Pregabalin undergoes negligible hepatic metabolism in humans and is eliminated from the systemic circulation primarily by renal excretion as the unchanged drug. Despite being a structural analogue to GABA, pregabalin does not show direct GABA-mimetic effects and has no effect on GABAergic mechanisms. Like gabapentin, pregabalin binds to the alpha2 delta1 subunit of the neuronal voltage-dependent calcium channel, thus reducing calcium influx into the nerve terminals and decreasing glutamate release. This mechanism of action appears to be responsible for the beneficial effects of pregabalin on epileptic seizures, neuropathic pain, and anxiety (which are its main indication). Despite being structurally related to gabapentin, pregabalin has shown considerably greater potency than gabapentin in seizure disorders.

Zonisamide

Zonisamide is a sulfonamide derivative chemically distinct from any of the previously established AEDs. Its antiepileptic action was discovered by chance in 1974, and it was approved for use in Japan long before it was licensed in Western Countries. Zonisamide is rapidly and completely absorbed, and peak concentrations are achieved usually within 2–7 hours. Bioavailability is close to 100% and protein binding is 30–60%. Zonisamide is metabolized by the CYP3A species of the cytochrome P450 system, followed by conjugation with glucuronic acid. The plasma half-life is 50–70 hours in monotherapy (lower in co-medication with enzyme-inducing drugs). Zonisamide exhibits first-order kinetics; its metabolites are not active and are excreted in the urine (about 35% of the drug is excreted unchanged). Zonisamide is a carbonic anhydrase inhibitor with a number of different properties, although the mechanism of action as an antiepileptic is thought to be through blockage of repetitive firing of voltage-sensitive sodium channels and reduction of voltage-sensitive T-type calcium currents. Zonisamide also binds to the benzodiazepine GABA-A receptor, has effects on excitatory glutaminergic transmission and acetylcholine metabolism, and inhibits dopamine turnover, but the relevance of these actions to its anticonvulsant action is unclear.

Eslicarbazepine

Eslicarbazepine (commercialized as a chemical compound called eslicarbazepine acetate) is a derivative of carbamazepine developed to improve tolerability without lowering efficacy of carbamazepine. Eslicarbazepine acetate is absorbed almost completely (at least 90%) from the gastrointestinal tract and is quickly metabolized to its active metabolite eslicarbazepine: Eslicarbazepine acetate is mostly undetectable after oral administration. Peak plasma levels of eslicarbazepine are reached after 1–4 hours, and plasma protein binding is less than 40%. Biological half-life is 10–20 hours, and steady-state concentrations are reached after 4–5 days. The drug is excreted mainly via the urine, of which two-thirds are in the form of eslicarbazepine and one-third in the form of eslicarbazepine glucuronide. Eslicarbazepine is thought to have the same mechanism of action as its racemate licarbazepine, a derivative of oxcarbazepine metabolism; both eslicarbazepine and licarbazepine are voltage-gated sodium channel blockers with anticonvulsant and mood-stabilizing effects.

Brivaracetam

Brivaracetam is a racetam derivative with antiepileptic properties developed after a major drug discovery programme aimed to identify selective, high-affinity SV2A ligands possessing anticonvulsant properties superior to levetiracetam and a better tolerability profile. Brivaracetam is rapidly and completely absorbed after oral administration. It exhibits linear pharmacokinetics over a wide dose range, has an elimination half-life of 7–8 hours, and has plasma protein binding of less than 20%. Brivaracetam is extensively metabolized (>90%), primarily via hydrolysis and secondarily through hydroxylation mediated by the liver enzyme CYP2C19. Brivaracetam is eliminated as urinary metabolites. The primary mechanism for brivaracetam anticonvulsant activity is believed to be binding to SV2A, which is thought to modulate exocytosis of neurotransmitters, thereby decreasing neuronal activation.

Other AEDs

Rufinamide

Rufinamide is a novel AED recently approved as adjunctive treatment for seizures associated with Lennox–Gastaut syndrome. Rufinamide is relatively well absorbed in the lower dose range, with approximately dose-proportional plasma concentrations at lower doses, but less than dose-proportional plasma concentrations at higher doses due to reduced oral bioavailability. Peak serum concentrations are reached within 4–6 hours. Rufinamide is not extensively bound to plasma proteins (34%) and its elimination half-life of 6–10 hours. Rufinamide is not a substrate of cytochrome P450 liver enzymes and is extensively metabolized in the liver via hydrolysis by carboxylesterases to a pharmacologically inactive metabolite, which is excreted in the urine. The mechanism of antiepileptic action of rufinamide is thought to be the prolongation of the inactive state of voltage-gated sodium channels.

Lacosamide

Lacosamide, formerly known as harkoseride, is a new AED recently approved as adjunctive therapy for focal seizures. Lacosamide is rapidly and completely absorbed after oral administration (oral bioavailability of about 100%). Peak plasma concentrations occur between 1 and 4 hours, and pharmacokinetics are linear. A small portion of lacosamide (less than 15%) is bound to plasma proteins and the plasma half-life is approximately 13 hours (range 12–16 hours). Metabolism is largely renal. Approximately 40% of the drug is excreted unchanged in the urine, while another 30% are recovered in the form of an inactive metabolite. The primary mode of action of lacosamide is thought to consist in enhancement of slow inactivation of voltage-gated sodium channels, a mechanism that differs from that of other sodium channel-blocking AEDs, which modulate fast inactivation.

Perampanel

Perampanel is one of the most interesting agents within the recently marketed newest AEDs (2012). Perampanel is rapidly absorbed after oral administration (time to maximum concentration 0.5–2.5 hours) and has a bioavailability of almost 100%. Perampanel is highly protein bound (about 95%) in plasma, and undergoes extensive hepatic metabolism (95%) to form 13 major inactive metabolites. The isoenzyme CYP3A4 is primarily considered to be involved in the hepatic metabolism of perampanel. Mean plasma half-life of perampanel in healthy adult volunteers is 105 hours. Elimination is both renal and faecal; the majority (about 70%) of an administered perampanel dose is excreted in faeces, whereas only 2% is excreted as unchanged perampanel in urine. Perampanel is a selective non-competitive antagonist of the AMPA glutamate receptor on postsynaptic neurons. This new agent showed high efficacy in a wide range of experimental epilepsy models and was licensed initially as adjunctive therapy for partial seizures, and subsequently for the treatment of primary generalized tonic-clonic seizures.

CHAPTER 3

Carbamazepine, oxcarbazepine, and eslicarbazepine

Carbamazepine is a first-generation antiepileptic drug (AED; Fig. 3.1) known with the proprietary brand name of Tegretol® (Novartis, Basel) in the UK and USA (Fig. 3.2). Oxcarbazepine is a second-generation AED (Fig. 3.1) supplied under the proprietary brand name of Trileptal® (Novartis, Basel) in the UK and USA (Fig. 3.3). Eslicarbazepine is a third-generation AED (Fig. 3.1) sold under the proprietary brand names of Zebinix® (Eisai, Hatfield) in the UK and Aptiom® (Sunovion, Marlborough, MS) in the USA (Fig. 3.4).

Preparations

Carbamazepine

Tablets
- Carbamazepine 100 mg (84-tab pack).
- Carbamazepine 200 mg (84-tab pack).
- Carbamazepine 400 mg (56-tab pack).

Modified-release tablets
- Carbamazepine 200 mg (56-tab pack).
- Carbamazepine 400 mg (56-tab pack).

Oral suspension
- Carbamazepine 20 mg/mL (300 mL).

Suppository
- Carbamazepine 125 mg (5-suppository pack).
- Carbamazepine 250 mg (5-suppository pack).

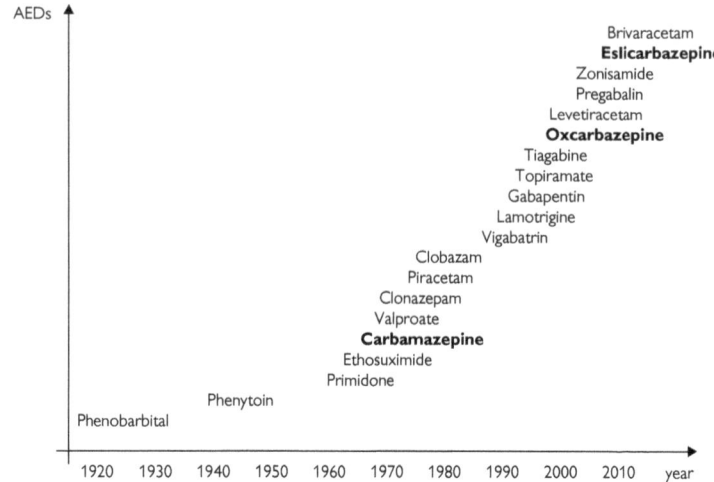

Fig. 3.1 Chronology of the clinical use of carbamazepine and its derivatives oxcarbazepine and eslicarbazepine

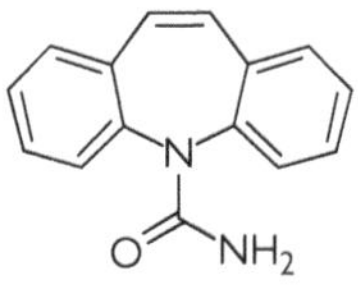

Fig. 3.2 Chemical structure of carbamazepine

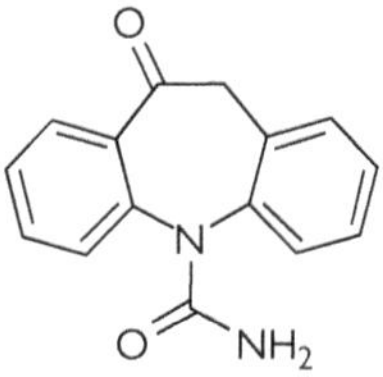

Fig. 3.3 Chemical structure of oxcarbazepine

CHAPTER 3

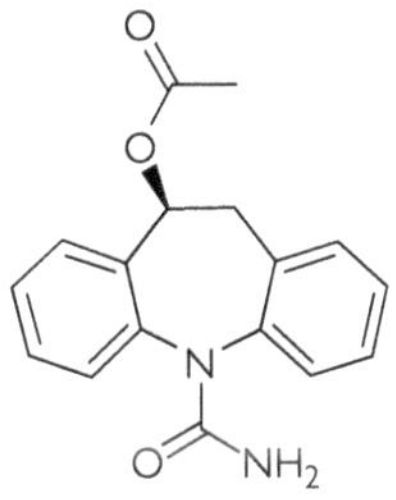

Fig. 3.4 Chemical structure of eslicarbazepine

Oxcarbazepine

Tablets
- Oxcarbazepine 150 mg (50-tab pack).
- Oxcarbazepine 300 mg (50-tab pack).
- Oxcarbazepine 600 mg (50-tab pack).

Oral suspension
- Oxcarbazepine 60 mg/mL (250 mL).

Eslicarbazepine

Tablets
- Eslicarbazepine 800 mg (30-tab pack).

Generic formulation

Carbamazepine

The Medicines and Healthcare Products Regulatory Agency/Commission on Human Medicines (MHRA/CHM) advice to minimize risk when switching patients with epilepsy between different manufacturers' products (including generic products):

- *Category 1*: doctors are advised to ensure that their patients are maintained on a specific manufacturer's product.

Oxcarbazepine and eslicarbazepine

MHRA/CHM advice to minimize risk when switching patients with epilepsy between different manufacturers' products (including generic products):

- *Category 2*: the need for continued supply of a particular manufacturer's product should be based on clinical judgment and consultation with the patient and/or carer, taking into account factors such as seizure frequency and treatment history.

Indications

Carbamazepine

Epilepsy: monotherapy and adjunctive therapy of focal and generalized seizures.

Recommendations

- *Seizure types*: first line (generalized tonic-clonic seizures, focal seizures), adjunctive (focal seizures), contraindicated (generalized tonic-clonic seizures if there are absence or myoclonic seizures, or if juvenile myoclonic epilepsy is suspected, tonic/atonic seizures, absence seizures, myoclonic seizures).
- *Epilepsy types*: first line (epilepsy with generalized tonic-clonic seizures only, benign epilepsy with centrotemporal spikes, Panayiotopoulos syndrome, late-onset childhood occipital epilepsy), adjunctive (benign epilepsy with centrotemporal spikes, Panayiotopoulos syndrome, late-onset childhood occipital epilepsy), contraindicated (absence syndromes, juvenile myoclonic epilepsy, idiopathic generalized epilepsy, Dravet syndrome, Lennox–Gastaut syndrome).
    - *Psychiatry*: prophylaxis of manic-depressive phases in patients with bipolar disorder unresponsive to lithium therapy; treatment of alcohol withdrawal symptoms (unlicensed).
    - *Neurology*: treatment of paroxysmal pain in trigeminal neuralgia and diabetic neuropathy (unlicensed).

Oxcarbazepine

Epilepsy: monotherapy and adjunctive therapy of focal and generalized seizures.

Recommendations summarized from NICE (2012)

- *Seizure types*: first line (generalized tonic-clonic seizures, focal seizures), adjunctive (focal seizures), contraindicated (generalized tonic-clonic seizures if there are absence or myoclonic seizures, or if juvenile myoclonic epilepsy is suspected, tonic/atonic seizures, absence seizures, myoclonic seizures).
- *Epilepsy types*: first line (epilepsy with generalized tonic-clonic seizures only, benign epilepsy with centrotemporal spikes, Panayiotopoulos

syndrome, late-onset childhood occipital epilepsy), adjunctive (benign epilepsy with centrotemporal spikes, Panayiotopoulos syndrome, late-onset childhood occipital epilepsy), contraindicated (absence syndromes, juvenile myoclonic epilepsy, idiopathic generalized epilepsy, Dravet syndrome, Lennox–Gastaut syndrome).

Eslicarbazepine

Epilepsy: monotherapy and adjunctive therapy of focal seizures.

Recommendations summarized from NICE (2012)
- *Seizure types*: adjunctive (focal seizures).

Dose titration

Carbamazepine

- *Epilepsy—immediate release*: 100–200 mg od/bd, increased by 100–200 mg every 14 days; usual maintenance 800–1200 mg daily, in divided doses (max. 2000 mg daily).
- *Epilepsy—prolonged release*: 50–200 mg bd, increased by 100–200 mg every 14 days; usual maintenance 800–1200 mg daily, divided into two doses (max. 2000 mg daily).
- *Bipolar disorder—immediate release*: 400 mg daily, in divided doses, increased by 100–200 mg every 14 days; usual maintenance 400–600 mg daily, in divided doses (max. 1600 mg daily).
- *Bipolar disorder—prolonged release*: 200 mg bd, increased by 100–200 mg every 14 days; usual maintenance 200–300 mg bd (max. 1600 mg daily).

If stopping carbamazepine, patients with bipolar disorder need to reduce the dose gradually over a period of at least 4 weeks.

Oxcarbazepine

300 mg bd, increased by 300–600 mg every 7 days; usual maintenance 600–2400 mg daily, in divided doses.

Eslicarbazepine

400 mg od, increased to 800 mg od after 1–2 weeks (max. 1200 mg od).

Plasma levels monitoring

Carbamazepine

Correlations between dosages and plasma levels of carbamazepine, as well as between plasma levels, and clinical efficacy or tolerability, are rather tenuous.

However, monitoring of the plasma levels (therapeutic range in the treatment of epilepsy 4–12 mg/L) may be useful in selected conditions, such as a dramatic increase in seizure frequency/verification of patient compliance, during pregnancy, in suspected absorption disorders, in suspected toxicity due to polymedication.

Oxcarbazepine

Plasma level monitoring of oxcarbazepine is not routinely warranted. Although correlations between dosage and plasma levels of oxcarbazepine, and between plasma levels and clinical efficacy or tolerability are rather tenuous, monitoring of the plasma levels may be useful to rule out non-compliance or in patients with changes in renal function, patients with concomitant use of liver enzyme-inducing drugs and during pregnancy.

Eslicarbazepine

Plasma level monitoring has a minimal role in the therapeutic use of eslicarbazepine due to the relatively predictable pharmacokinetics of the drug.

Cautions

Carbamazepine

- Patients with a history of hepatic porphyrias.
- Patients with a history of bone marrow depression.
- Patients with atrioventricular block.
- Patients with a history of haematological reactions to other drugs.
- Patients with susceptibility to angle-closure glaucoma.
- Patients with skin reactions.
- Patients with cardiac disease.
- Patients with absence and myoclonic seizures.

Oxcarbazepine

- Patients with acute porphyrias.
- Patients with cardiac disease.
- Patients with hyponatraemia.

Eslicarbazepine

- Elderly patients.
- Patients with hyponatraemia.
- Patients with prolonged PR interval.

Adverse effects

Carbamazepine

Carbamazepine can be associated with adverse effects at the level of the nervous system and other systems (Table 3.1).

Some adverse effects (mainly affecting the nervous system) are dose-dependent and may be dose-limiting. The incidence of these adverse effects (higher at the start of treatment and in the elderly) can be reduced by offering a modified-release preparation or altering the timing of medication. Although the

Table 3.1 Estimated frequency of adverse effects of carbamazepine

Very common (>1 in 10 patients on carbamazepine)	
Nervous system • ataxia • dizziness • tiredness	*Other systems* • nausea and vomiting • leucopenia • skin rash
Common (>1 in 100 patients on carbamazepine)	
Nervous system • headache • diplopia	*Other systems* • dry mouth • hyponatraemia • oedema • thrombocytopenia • weight gain
Uncommon (>1 in 1000 patients on carbamazepine)	
Nervous system • involuntary movements • nystagmus	*Other systems* • constipation • diarrhoea
Rare (>1 in 10,000 patients on carbamazepine)	
Nervous system • agitation • aggression • confusion • dysarthria • depression • hallucinations • paraesthesias • restlessness • weakness	*Other systems* • abdominal pain • anorexia • arrhythmias • delayed multi-organ hypersensitivity disorder • hypertension • hypotension • jaundice • lupus erythematosus-like syndrome • lymphadenopathy

(continued)

Table 3.1 Continued	
Very rare (<1 in 10,000 patients on carbamazepine)	
Nervous system • hearing disorders • psychosis • taste disturbance	*Other systems* • acne • alopecia • alterations in skin pigmentation • anaemia • angle-closure glaucoma • aseptic meningitis • conjunctivitis • dyspnoea • gynaecomastia and galactorrhoea • hirsutism • impotence, loss of libido and impaired male fertility • kidney failure • liver failure • muscle pain and spasms • ostomalacia and osteoporosis • photosensitivity • purpura • severe skin reaction (Stevens-Johnson syndrome)* • stomatitis • sweating • thromboembolism and thrombophlebitis • toxic epidermal necrolysis • urinary frequency or retention

*Before deciding to initiate treatment, patients of Han Chinese and Thai origin should, whenever possible, be screened for HLA-B*1502, as this allele strongly predicts the risk of severe carbamazepine-associated Stevens–Johnson syndrome.

manufacturer recommends blood counts, and hepatic and renal functions tests, evidence of practical value is uncertain.

Oxcarbazepine

Oxcarbazepine can be associated with adverse effects at the level of the nervous system and other systems (Table 3.2).

Eslicarbazepine

Eslicarbazepine can be associated with adverse effects at the level of the nervous system and other systems (Table 3.3).

Table 3.2 Estimated frequency of adverse effects of oxcarbazepine

Very common (>1 in 10 patients on oxcarbazepine)	
Nervous system • diplopia • dizziness • headache • tiredness	*Other systems* • nausea and vomiting

Common (>1 in 100 patients on oxcarbazepine)	
Nervous system • agitation • amnesia • anxiety • ataxia • confusion • depression • drowsiness • nystagmus • tremor • weakness	*Other systems* • abdominal pain • acne • alopecia • constipation • diarrhoea • hyponatraemia • skin rash

Uncommon (>1 in 1,000 patients on oxcarbazepine)	
Nervous system	*Other systems* • leucopenia • urticaria

Rare (>1 in 10,000 patients on oxcarbazepine)	
Nervous system	*Other systems*

Very rare (<1 in 10,000 patients on oxcarbazepine)	
Nervous system	*Other systems* • arrhythmias • atrioventricular block • delayed multi-organ hypersensitivity disorder • hepatitis • lupus erythematosus-like syndrome • pancreatitis • severe skin reaction (Stevens-Johnson syndrome)* • thrombocytopenia • toxic epidermal necrolysis

*Before deciding to initiate treatment, patients of Han Chinese and Thai origin should, whenever possible, be screened for HLA-B*1502, as this allele strongly predicts the risk of severe oxcarbazepine-associated Stevens–Johnson syndrome.

Table 3.3 Estimated frequency of adverse effects of eslicarbazepine

Very common (>1 in 10 patients on eslicarbazepine)	
Nervous system • dizziness • tiredness	*Other systems*
Common (>1 in 100 patients on eslicarbazepine)	
Nervous system • ataxia • diplopia • headache • insomnia • tremor • weakness	*Other systems* • decreased appetite • diarrhoea • hyponatraemia • nausea and vomiting • skin rash
Uncommon (>1 in 1000 patients on eslicarbazepine)	
Nervous system • agitation • amnesia • anxiety • confusion • depression • disaesthesia • dysarthria • hyperactivity • movement disorders • nystagmus • parosmia • tinnitus	*Other systems* • abdominal pain • alopecia • anaemia • bradycardia • chest pain • constipation • dehydration • dry mouth • electrolyte imbalances • epistaxis • gingival hyperplasia • hypertension • hyponatraemia • hypotension • hypothyroidism • liver problems • malaise • myalgia • peripheral oedema • stomatitis • urinary tract infection • weight loss
Rare (>1 in 10,000 patients on eslicarbazepine)	
Nervous system	*Other systems*
Very rare (<1 in 10,000 patients on eslicarbazepine)	
Nervous system	*Other systems* • leucopenia • pancreatitis • thrombocytopenia

Rare adverse reactions, such as bone marrow depression, anaphylactic reactions, severe cutaneous reactions (e.g. Stevens–Johnson syndrome), systemic lupus erythematosus, or serious cardiac arrhythmias did not occur during the placebo-controlled studies of the epilepsy programme with eslicarbazepine acetate. However, they have been reported with carbamazepine and oxcarbazepine. Therefore, their occurrence after treatment with eslicarbazepine acetate cannot be excluded.

Interactions

Carbamazepine

With AEDs

- Plasma concentration of carbamazapine is increased by vigabatrin, whereas plasma concentration of the active metabolite carbamazepine 10,11-epoxide is increased by primidone and valproate (reduce carbamazepine dose to avoid increased risk of toxicity).
- Plasma concentration of carbamazepine is reduced by cytochrome P450 3A4 inducers (including eslicarbazepine, oxcarbazepine, phenobarbital, phenytoin, primidone, and, possibly, clonazepam).
- Carbamazepine is a cytochrome P450 3A4 inducer and can decrease the plasma concentration of clobazam, clonazepam, ethosuximide, lamotrigine, oxcarbazepine, primidone, tiagabine, topiramate, valproate, and zonisamide.
- Co-administration of levetiracetam has been reported to increase carbamazepine-induced toxicity; cross-sensitivity has been reported with oxcarbazepine and phenytoin.

With other drugs

- Plasma concentration of carbamazepine is reduced by cytochrome P450 3A4 inducers aminophylline, cisplatin, doxorubicin, St John's wort (*Hypericum perforatum*), isotretinoin, rifampicin, and theophylline (consider increasing the dose of carbamazepine).
- Plasma concentration of carbamazepine is increased by cytochrome P450 3A4 inhibitors: acetazolamide, azoles (antifungals), cimetidine, ciprofloxacine, danazol, dextropropoxyphene, diltiazem, fluoxetine, fluvoxamine, isoniazid, loratadine, macrolide antibiotics, olanzapine, omeprazole, paroxetine, protease inhibitors (antivirals), trazodone, and verapamil. Plasma concentration of the active metabolite carbamazepine-10,11-epoxide is increased by progabide, quetiapine, valnoctamide, and valpromide.
- Carbamazepine is a cytochrome P450 3A4 inducer and can decrease the plasma concentration of albendazole, alprazolam, aprepitant, aripiprazole,

atorvastatin, bromperidol, buprenorphine, bupropion, calcium channel blockers (e.g. felodipine), cerivastatin, ciclosporin, citalopram, clozapine, corticosteroids (e.g. prednisolone, dexamethasone), cyclophosphamide, digoxin, doxycycline, everolimus, haloperidol, hormonal contraceptives (oestrogens and progesterones), imatinib, itraconazole, ivabradine, lapatinib, levothyroxine, lovastatin, methadone, mianserin, olanzapine, oral anticoagulants (e.g. warfarin), paliperidone, paracetamol (acetaminophen), protease inhibitors (antivirals), quetiapine, rifabutin, risperidone, sertraline, simvastatin, tacrolimus, tadalafil, temsirolimus, theophylline, tramadol, trazodone, tricyclic antidepressants, voriconazole, and sirolimus.

With alcohol/food

- Drinking alcohol may affect patients more than usual; eating grapefruit, or drinking grapefruit juice, may increase chance of experiencing adverse effects.

Oxcarbazepine

With AEDs

- Strong inducers of cytochrome P450 enzymes (i.e. carbamazepine, phenytoin, phenobarbital) have been shown to decrease the plasma levels of oxcarbazepine's pharmacologically active metabolite.
- Oxcarbazepine and its pharmacologically active metabolite are weak inducers of the cytochrome P450 enzymes CYP3A4 and CYP3A5 responsible for the metabolism of a other AEDs (e.g. carbamazepine) resulting in a lower plasma concentration of these medicinal products.
- Concomitant therapy of oxcarbazepine and lamotrigine has been associated with an increased risk of adverse events (nausea, somnolence, dizziness, and headache).

With other drugs

- Oxcarbazepine and its pharmacologically active metabolite are weak inducers of the cytochrome P450 enzymes CYP3A4 and CYP3A5 responsible for the metabolism of a large number of drugs, for example, immunosuppressants (e.g. ciclosporin, tacrolimus) and oral contraceptives (see carbamazepine's interactions).

With alcohol/food

- Caution should be exercised if alcohol is taken in combination with oxcarbazepine, due to a possible additive sedative effect.
- There are no specific foods that must be excluded from diet when taking oxcarbazepine.

Eslicarbazepine

With AEDs

- Concomitant administration of eslicarbazepine and carbamazepine or phenytoin can result in a decrease in exposure to the active metabolite of eslicarbazepine, most likely caused by an induction of glucuronidation. therefore, the dose of eslicarbazepine may need to be increased if used concomitantly with carbamazepine.
- Concomitant administration of eslicarbazepine and phenytoin can result in an increase in exposure to phenytoin, most likely caused by an inhibition of CYP2C19.
- Concomitant use of eslicarbazepine with oxcarbazepine is not recommended because this may cause overexposure to the active metabolites.

With other drugs

- Concomitant administration of eslicarbazepine and combined oral contraceptive, simvastatin, rosuvastatin, and warfarin results in a decrease in systemic exposure to levonorgestrel and ethinylestradiol, simvastatin, rosuvastatin, and warfarin, most probably caused by an induction of CYP3A4.
- Based on a structural relationship of eslicarbazepine to tricyclic antidepressants, an interaction between eslicarbazepine and monoamino oxidase inhibitors is theoretically possible.

With alcohol/food

- There are no known specific interactions between alcohol and eslicarbazepine, and there are no specific foods that must be excluded from the diet when taking eslicarbazepine.

Special populations

Carbamazepine

Hepatic impairment

- Metabolism impaired in advanced liver disease.

Renal impairment

- Use with caution.

Pregnancy

- Developmental disorders and malformations (including spina bifida), as well as other congenital anomalies (including craniofacial defects, such as cleft lip/palate, cardiovascular malformations, hypospadias, and anomalies involving various body systems) have been reported in association with the use of carbamazepine during pregnancy. In women of childbearing age carbamazepine should, wherever possible, be prescribed as monotherapy, because the incidence of congenital abnormalities in the offspring of women treated with a combination of antiepileptic drugs is greater (especially if valproate is part of the polytherapy).

- Pregnant women with epilepsy should be treated with minimum effective doses of carbamazepine and monitoring of plasma levels is recommended (aiming at the lower side of the therapeutic range, as there is evidence to suggest that the risk of malformation with carbamazepine may be dose-dependent).
- Should a woman on carbamazepine decide to breastfeed, the infant should be monitored for possible adverse effects, as carbamazepine can be excreted in considerable amounts in breastmilk, which in combination with slow infantile elimination can result in plasma concentrations at which pharmacological effects occur. Since there have been reports of cholestatic hepatitis in neonates exposed to carbamazepine during antenatal and or during breastfeeding, breastfed infants of mothers treated with carbamazepine should be carefully observed for adverse hepatobiliary effects.

Oxcarbazepine

Hepatic impairment

- Mild to moderate hepatic impairment does not affect the pharmacokinetics of oxcarbazepine and its active metabolite. Oxcarbazepine has not been studied in patients with severe hepatic impairment.

Renal impairment

- Dose adjustment (halve initial dose and increase according to response at intervals of at least 1 week) is recommended in patients with renal impairment and lower creatinine clearance.

Pregnancy

- Data on oxcarbazepine associated with congenital malformation are limited. There is no increase in the total rate of malformations with oxcarbazepine, compared with the rate observed in the general population. However, a moderate teratogenic risk cannot be completely excluded.
- If women receiving oxcarbazepine become pregnant or plan to become pregnant, the use of this drug should be carefully re-evaluated. Minimum effective doses should be given, and monotherapy whenever possible should be preferred at least during the first 3 months of pregnancy.

- During pregnancy, an effective antiepileptic oxcarbazepine treatment must not be interrupted, since the aggravation of the illness is detrimental to both the mother and the foetus.
- Oxcarbazepine and its active metabolite are excreted in human breastmilk. As the effects on the infant exposed to oxcarbazepine by this route are unknown, oxcarbazepine should not be used during breast-feeding.

Eslicarbazepine

Hepatic impairment

- No dose adjustment is recommended in patients with mild to moderate hepatic impairment.
- The pharmacokinetics of eslicarbazepine has not been evaluated in patients with severe hepatic impairment.

Renal impairment

- Dose adjustment (reduce initial dose to 400 mg every other day for 2 weeks, then 400 mg od) is recommended in patients with renal impairment and lower creatinine clearance.

Pregnancy

- There are no data from the use of eslicarbazepine in pregnant women. If women receiving eslicarbazepine become pregnant or plan to become pregnant, the use of eslicarbazepine should be carefully re-evaluated. Minimum effective doses should be given and monotherapy, whenever possible, should be preferred, at least during the first 3 months of pregnancy.
- It is unknown whether eslicarbazepine acetate is excreted in human milk. As a risk to the breastfed child cannot be excluded, breastfeeding should be discontinued during treatment with eslicarbazepine

Behavioural and cognitive effects in patients with epilepsy

Carbamazepine

Carbamazepine is characterized by a good behavioural and cognitive profile in patients with epilepsy. Overall, adverse psychiatric effects (especially irritation, agitation, depression) are rarely reported in this patient population. Moderate cognitive problems affecting attention, memory, and language have occasionally been reported (especially at high doses).

Oxcarbazepine

Similarly to carbamazepine, oxcarbazepine is generally considered to pose a low risk for adverse psychiatric effects (especially emotional lability, insomnia, abnormal thinking—usually occurring at high dosages) in patients with epilepsy.

Moderate cognitive problems affecting attention and concentration have occasionally been reported (especially at high doses).

Eslicarbazepine

For this third-generation agent, clinical experience is still limited, and little is known about its positive and negative psychotropic properties, and their implications for the management of behavioural symptoms in patients with epilepsy.

Psychiatric use

Carbamazepine

Carbamazepine was approved as a treatment for acute mania in 2004, decades after it was recognized as an effective alternative to lithium in the management of bipolar illness. Data from open-label trials suggest that carbamazepine is effective in the prophylaxis of bipolar disorder or acute mania, but may be less effective than valproate or lithium. However, carbamazepine has been suggested to be a better alternative for atypical manifestations of bipolar disorder, such as rapid cycling course, mood-incongruent delusions, or in the presence of other co-morbid psychiatric or neurological conditions. Carbamazepine may also be effective in unipolar depression, whereas its utility in schizophrenia is uncertain. In rarer cases, carbamazepine has been used to treat aggressive behaviour and to facilitate sedatives/alcohol withdrawal, but there is no solid evidence to date to establish its efficacy in this domain. To summarize, evidence is strongest to support the mood stabilizing properties of carbamazepine (Fig. 3.5).

Oxcarbazepine

Oxcarbazepine's principal use in patients with psychiatric disorder is the treatment of bipolar disorder (mania), although there are no approved indications in psychiatry. Oxcarbazepine has been proposed as a potential option for add-on therapy in the treatment of bipolar disorder, although it remains to be determined whether oxcarbazepine is effective in the acute treatment of bipolar depression or the maintenance treatment of bipolar disorder. Preliminary evidence suggests that oxcarbazepine may exert beneficial effects on behavioural disorders, particularly impulsive aggression. There is also evidence for the potential usefulness of oxcarbazepine in obsessive-compulsive disorder and anxiety disorders (panic disorder, post-traumatic stress disorder). Other potential off-label uses are alcohol withdrawal and dependence, benzodiazepine withdrawal, and cocaine abuse/dependence (Fig. 3.6).

Eslicarbazepine

For this third-generation agent, clinical experience is still limited and little is known about its positive and negative psychotropic properties, and their implications for the management of behavioural symptoms in patients with epilepsy.

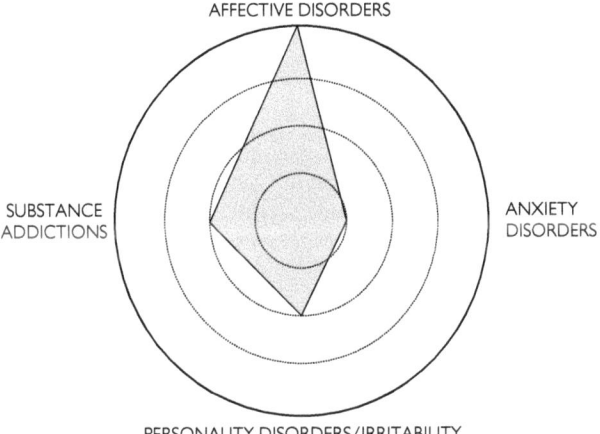

Fig. 3.5 Level of evidence supporting the psychiatric use of carbamazepine in patients with behavioural symptoms

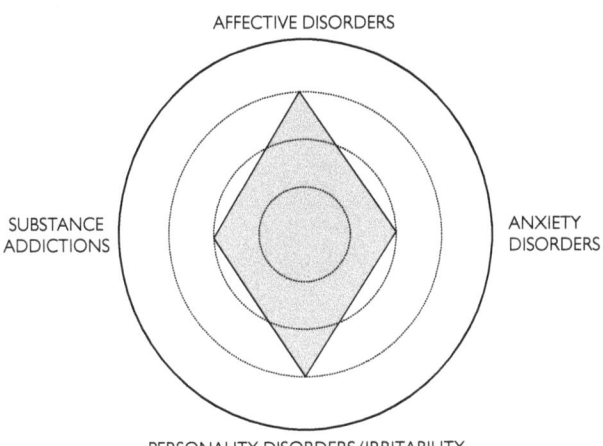

Fig. 3.6 Level of evidence supporting the psychiatric use of oxcarbazepine in patients with behavioural symptoms

Table 3.4 Overall rating of carbamazepine	
Antiepileptic indications	☺☺
Interactions in polytherapy	☺
Behavioural tolerability	☺☺☺
Psychiatric use	☺☺☺
Key: ☺☺☺ = very good; ☺☺ = good; ☺ = acceptable.	

Overall rating

Carbamazepine

Carbamazepine is characterized by a good range of antiepileptic indications, with acceptable risk of interactions in polytherapy. It has a very good behavioural tolerability profile and widespread psychiatric use (Table 3.4).

Oxcarbazepine

Oxcarbazepine is characterized by a good range of antiepileptic indications, with acceptable risk of interactions in polytherapy. It has a very good behavioural tolerability profile and potential for widespread psychiatric use (Table 3.5).

Table 3.5 Overall rating of oxcarbazepine	
Antiepileptic indications	☺☺
Interactions in polytherapy	☺
Behavioural tolerability	☺☺☺
Psychiatric use	☺☺
Key: ☺☺☺ = very good; ☺☺ = good; ☺ = acceptable.	

CHAPTER 4

Clonazepam and clobazam

Clonazepam

Clonazepam is a first-generation antiepileptic drug (AED; Fig. 4.1) known under the proprietary brand name of Klonopin® (Roche, Basel) in the USA (Fig. 4.2).

Clobazam

Clobazam is a first-generation AED (Fig. 4.1) known under the proprietary brand name of Frisium® (Sanofi, Paris) in the UK and Onfi® (Lundbeck, Copenhagen) in the USA (Fig. 4.3).

Preparations

Clonazepam

Tablets
- Clonazepam 0.5 mg (100-tab pack).
- Clonazepam 2 mg (100-tab pack).

Oral solution
- Clonazepam 0.1 mg/mL (150 mL).
- Clonazepam 0.4 mg/mL (150 mL).

Clobazam

Tablets
- Clobazam 10 mg (30-tab pack).

Oral suspension
- Clobazam 1 mg/mL (150 mL).
- Clobazam 2 mg/mL (150 mL).

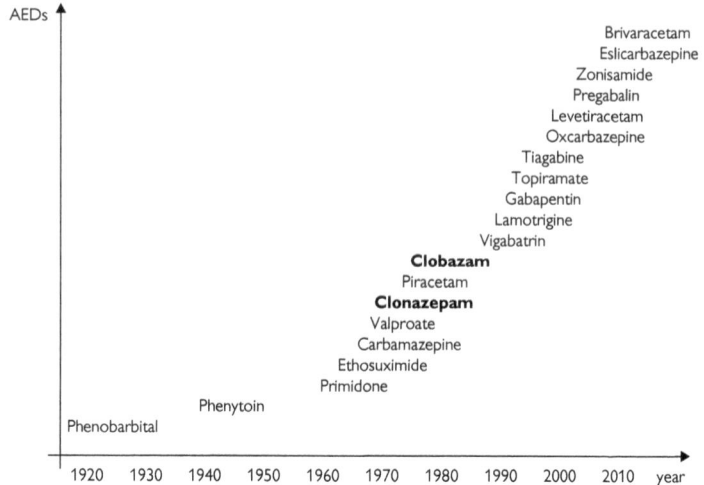

Fig. 4.1 Chronology of the clinical use of benzodiazepines clonazepam and clobazam

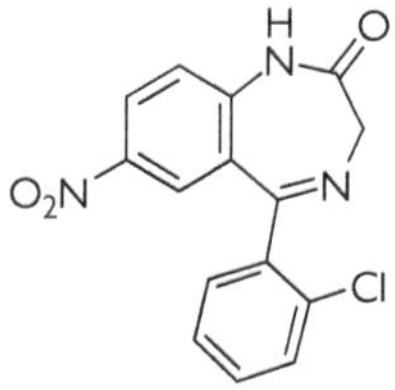

Fig. 4.2 Chemical structure of clonazepam

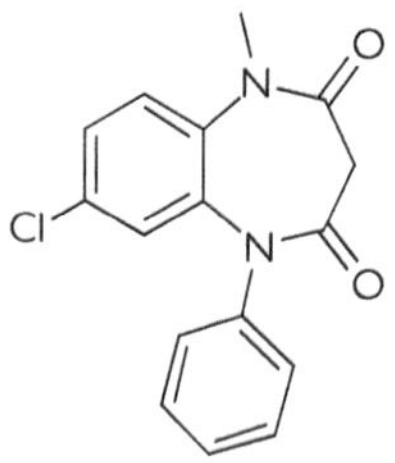

Fig. 4.3 Chemical structure of clobazam

Generic formulation

Clobazam, clonazepam

MHRA/CHM advice to minimize risk when switching patients with epilepsy between different manufacturers' products (including generic products):

- *Category 2*: the need for continued supply of a particular manufacturer's product should be based on clinical judgment, and consultation with the patient and/or carer, taking into account factors such as seizure frequency and treatment history.

Indications

Clonazepam

Epilepsy: monotherapy and adjunctive therapy of focal and generalized seizures.

Recommendations summarized from NICE (2012)
- *Seizure types*: on referral to tertiary care (absence seizures, myoclonic seizures).
- *Epilepsy types*: on referral to tertiary care (absence syndromes, juvenile myoclonic epilepsy, idiopathic generalized epilepsy).

Clobazam

Epilepsy: adjunctive therapy of focal and generalized seizures.

Recommendations summarized from NICE (2012)
- *Seizure types*: adjunctive (generalized tonic-clonic seizures, focal seizures), on referral to tertiary care (absence seizures, myoclonic seizures).
- *Epilepsy types*: adjunctive (epilepsy with generalized tonic-clonic seizures only), on referral to tertiary care (absence syndromes, juvenile myoclonic epilepsy, idiopathic generalized epilepsy):
  - *Psychiatry*—short-term relief (2–4 weeks) of severe, disabling, or unacceptably distressing anxiety, occurring alone or in association with insomnia, or short-term psychosomatic, organic, or psychotic illness (adjunctive treatment in patients with psychotic illness).

Dose titration

Clonazepam

Epilepsy: 1 mg nocte for 4 days, then increased over 2–4 weeks; usual maintenance dose 4–8 mg nocte or divided into 3 or 4 doses.

Clobazam

- *Epilepsy—adjunctive therapy*: 20–30 mg daily (max. 60 mg daily in divided doses).
- *Anxiety (short-term use)*: 20–30 mg nocte or in divided doses (max. 60 mg daily, in divided doses).

The effectiveness of clonazepam and clobazam may decrease significantly after weeks or months of continuous therapy.

Plasma levels monitoring

Routine measurement of plasma concentrations of clonazepam and clobazam is not usually justified, because the target concentration ranges are arbitrary and often vary between individuals. However, plasma drug concentrations may be measured in case of suspected non-compliance or toxicity.

Cautions

Clonazepam

- Patients with depression/suicidal ideation.
- Patients with brain damage.
- Patients with cerebellar/spinal ataxia.
- Patients with acute porphyrias.
- Patients with airways obstruction.

Clobazam

- Patients with dependent/avoidant/obsessive–compulsive personality disorder (may increase risk of dependence).
- Patients with organic brain damage.
- Patients with muscle weakness.

Adverse effects

Clonazepam

Clonazepam can be associated with adverse effects at the level of the nervous system and other systems (Table 4.1).

Clobazam

Clobazam can be associated with adverse effects at the level the nervous system and other systems (Table 4.2).

Table 4.1 Estimated frequency of adverse effects of clonazepam	
Very common or common (>1 in 10 or >1 in 100 patients on clonazepam)	
Nervous system • amnesia • ataxia • confusion • dependence • dizziness • drowsiness • fatigue • nystagmus • poor concentration • restlessness	*Other systems* • muscle hypotonia
Uncommon (>1 in 1000 patients on clonazepam)	
Nervous system	*Other systems*
Rare (>1 in 10,000 patients on clonazepam)	
Nervous system • aggression • anxiety • dysarthria • headache • suicidal ideation • visual disturbances (on long-term treatment)	*Other systems* • alopecia (reversible) • blood disorders • gastro-intestinal symptoms • pruritus • respiratory depression • sexual dysfunction • skin pigmentation changes • urinary incontinence • urticaria
Very rare (<1 in 10,000 patients on clonazepam)	
Nervous system • worsening of seizures	*Other systems*

Interactions

Clonazepam

With AEDs

Plasma concentration of clonazepam can be reduced by carbamazepine, phenobarbital, phenytoin, and primidone.

With other drugs

- Plasma concentration of clonazepam is decreased by rifampicin and can be reduced by theophylline.

Table 4.2 Estimated frequency of adverse effects of clobazam

Very common or common (>1 in 10 or >1 in 100 patients on clobazam)

Nervous system	Other systems
• amnesia • ataxia • confusion • dependence • drowsiness • lightheadedness • paradoxical increase in aggression	• muscle weakness

Uncommon (>11 in 1000 patients on clobazam)

Nervous system	Other systems
• changes in libido • dizziness • dysarthria • headache • tremor • vertigo • visual disturbances	• changes in salivation • gastro-intestinal symptoms • gynaecomastia • hypotension • urinary incontinence/retention

Rare (>1 in 10,000 patients on clobazam)

Nervous system	Other systems
	• blood disorders • jaundice • respiratory depression • skin reactions

Very rare (<1 in 10,000 patients on clobazam)

Nervous system	Other systems

- Plasma concentration of clonazepam is increased by cimetidine, disulfiram, fluvoxamine, and ritonavir
- There is an increased risk of prolonged sedation and respiratory depression when clonazepam is given with amprenavir.
- There are enhanced hypotensive and sedative effects when clonazepam is given with alpha-blockers or moxonidine.
- There is an enhanced hypotensive effect when clonazepam is given with ACE inhibitors, adrenergic neurone blockers, angiotensin-II receptor antagonists, beta-blockers, calcium channel blockers, clonidine, diazoxide, diuretics, hydralazine, methyldopa, minoxidil, nitrates, or nitroprusside.
- There is an increased sedative effect when clonazepam is given with general anaesthetics, tricyclic antidepressants, antihistamines, antipsychotics, baclofen, lofexidine, mirtazapine, nabilone, opioid analgesics, tizanidine.
- Clonazepam may possibly antagonize the effects of levodopa.

Clobazam

With AEDs

Phenytoin and carbamazepine may cause an increase in the metabolic conversion of clobazam to the active metabolite N-desmethyl clobazam.

With other drugs

- With administration of clobazam (especially at higher doses), an enhancement of the central depressive effect may occur in cases of concomitant use with antipsychotics, hypnotics, anxiolytics/sedatives, antidepressant agents, narcotic analgesics, anticonvulsant drugs, anaesthetics, and sedative antihistamines.
- If clobazam is used concomitantly with narcotic analgesics, possible euphoria may be enhanced (possibly leading to increased psychological dependence).
- The effects of muscle relaxants, analgesics and nitrous oxide may be enhanced by concomitant use of clobazam.
- Dosage adjustment of clobazam may be necessary when co-administered with strong (e.g. fluconazole, fluvoxamine, ticlopidine) or moderate (e.g. omeprazole) CYP2C19 inhibitors, which may result in increased exposure to N-desmethyl clobazam, the active metabolite of clobazam.
- Dose adjustment of drugs metabolized by CYP2D6 (e.g. dextromethorphan, nebivolol, paroxetine, and pimozide) may be necessary, as clobazam is a weak CYP2D6 inhibitor.

With alcohol/food

There is an increased sedative effect when clonazepam or clobazam are given with alcohol, and it is recommended that patients abstain from drinking alcohol during treatment with these drugs.

Special populations

Hepatic impairment

- Start with smaller initial dose or reduce maintenance dose.
- Avoid in severe impairment.

Renal impairment

Start with smaller dose in significant impairment.

Pregnancy

- As a precautionary measure, it is preferable to avoid the use of clonazepam and clobazam during pregnancy. Clonazepam and clobazam should be used during pregnancy only if the potential benefit justifies the potential risk to the foetus.

- Administration of clonazepam and clobazam in the last trimester of pregnancy or during labour can result in hypothermia, hypotonia, respiratory depression, and feeding difficulties in the neonate.
- Infants born to mothers who have taken clonazepam and clobazam during the later stages of pregnancy may develop physical dependence, and may be at risk for developing withdrawal symptoms in the postnatal period.
- Clonazepam and clobazam, like all benzodiazepines, are present in milk and should be avoided if possible during breastfeeding.

Behavioural and cognitive effects in patients with epilepsy

Clonazepam

Behavioural effects include sleepiness, poor coordination, and agitation with paradoxical aggression/disinhibition (usually dose-dependent). Long-term use may result in tolerance, dependence, and withdrawal symptoms if stopped abruptly. In addition to seizure exacerbation, abrupt discontinuation of benzodiazepines can be accompanied by changes in mental status, including anxiety, agitation, confusion, depression, psychosis, and delirium. Dependence occurs in one-third of patients who take clonazepam for longer than 4 weeks. Moreover, clonazepam may aggravate symptoms in patients who are depressed. Benzodiazepines are more frequently associated with adverse cognitive effects than most other AEDs. Among these, anterograde amnesia has been reported in patients treated with clonazepam (mainly at high doses).

Clobazam

Behavioural effects include sleepiness, poor coordination, and agitation with paradoxical aggression/disinhibition (usually dose-dependent). Long-term use may result in tolerance, dependence, and withdrawal symptoms if stopped abruptly. In addition to seizure exacerbation, abrupt discontinuation of benzodiazepines can be accompanied by changes in mental status, including anxiety, agitation, confusion, depression, psychosis, and delirium. Benzodiazepines are more frequently associated with adverse cognitive effects than most other AEDs. Among cognitive domains, attention and language appear to be more significantly affected in patients treated with clobazam (mainly at high doses).

Psychiatric use

Clonazepam

Clonazepam has been found to be effective in the short-term treatment of anxiety disorders, including generalized anxiety disorder, social phobia, and panic disorder. Catatonia, alcohol withdrawal, and insomnia are other common indications supported by evidence. Clonazepam is also sometimes used for the treatment of

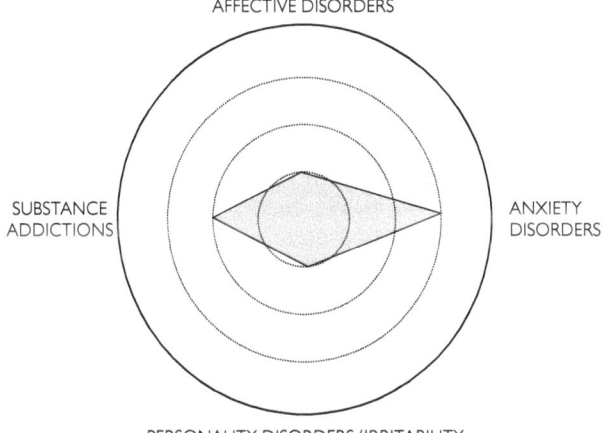

Fig. 4.4 Level of evidence supporting the psychiatric use of clonazepam and clobazam in patients with behavioural symptoms

acute mania, or psychosis-induced aggression and agitation (adjunctive treatment for bipolar disorder and schizophrenia) (Fig. 4.4).

Clobazam

In addition to its role as an AED, clobazam has an indication for short-term relief (2–4 weeks) of acute anxiety in patients who have not responded to other drugs, with or without insomnia, and without uncontrolled clinical depression (Fig. 4.4).

Overall rating

Clonazepam and clobazam are characterized by a few antiepileptic indications, with a good interaction profile in polytherapy. Both drugs have an acceptable behavioural tolerability profile and a good range of psychiatric uses (Table 4.3).

Table 4.3 Overall rating of clonazepam and clobazam	
Antiepileptic indications	☺
Interactions in polytherapy	☺ ☺
Behavioural tolerability	☺
Psychiatric use	☺ ☺
Key: ☺ ☺ ☺ = very good; ☺ ☺ = good; ☺ = acceptable.	

CHAPTER 5

Ethosuximide

Ethosuximide is a first-generation antiepileptic drug (AED; Fig. 5.1) known under the proprietary brand name of Zarontin® (Pfizer, New York, NY) in the UK (oral solution) and USA (Fig. 5.2).

Preparations

Capsule
Ethosuximide 250 mg (56-cap pack).

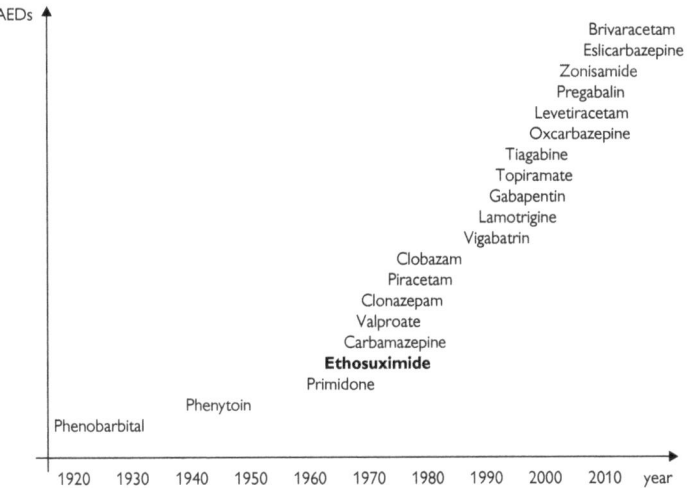

Fig. 5.1 Chronology of the clinical use of ethosuximide

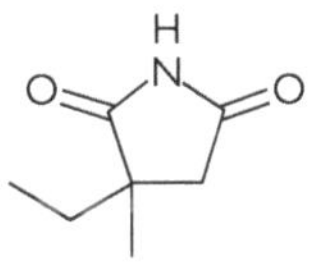

Fig. 5.2 Chemical structure of ethosuximide

Oral solution
Ethosuximide 50 mg/mL (200 mL).

Generic formulation
MHRA/CHM advice to minimize risk when switching patients with epilepsy between different manufacturers' products (including generic products):

- *Category 3*: it is usually unnecessary to ensure that patients are maintained on a specific manufacturer's product unless there are specific concerns, such as patient anxiety and risk of confusion/dosing error.

Indications
Epilepsy: monotherapy and adjunctive therapy of absence seizures; adjunctive therapy of generalized tonic-clonic seizures.

Recommendations summarized from NICE (2012)
- *Seizure types*: first line (absence seizures), adjunctive (absence seizures).
- *Epilepsy types*: first line (absence syndromes), adjunctive (absence syndromes).

Dose titration
250 mg bd, then increased in steps of 250 mg every 5–7 days; usual maintenance 1000–1500 mg daily, divided into two doses (max. 2000 mg daily).

Plasma levels monitoring
Monitoring ethosuximide plasma levels can be useful in selected cases, although the evidence for a therapeutic plasma range is limited (suggested therapeutic plasma concentrations 40–100 mg/L) and a toxic limit has not been consistently defined.

Cautions
Patients with acute porphyrias.

Adverse effects
Ethosuximide can be associated with adverse effects at the level the nervous system and other systems (Table 5.1).

Table 5.1 Estimated frequency of adverse effects of ethosuximide

Very common (>1 in 10 patients on ethosuximide)	
Nervous system	Other systems
Common (>1 in 100 patients on ethosuximide)	
Nervous system	Other systems • abdominal pain • anorexia • diarrhoea • gastro-intestinal disturbances • nausea and vomiting • weight loss
Uncommon (>1 in 1,000 patients on ethosuximide)	
Nervous system • aggression • ataxia • dizziness • drowsiness • euphoria • fatigue • headache • impaired concentration • irritability	Other systems • hiccup
Rare (>1 in 10,000 patients on ethosuximide)	
Nervous system: • depression • dyskinesia • increased libido • myopia • photophobia • psychosis • sleep disturbances	Other systems: • gingival hypertrophy • rash • tongue swelling • vaginal bleeding
Very rare (<1 in 10,000 patients on ethosuximide)	
Nervous system	Other systems

Interactions

With AEDs

- Plasma concentration of ethosuximide is reduced by the glucuronidation inducers carbamazepine, phenytoin, phenobarbital, and primidone.

- Plasma concentration of ethosuximide has been reported to be both increased and decreased by valproate.
- Ethosuximide can raise serum levels of phenytoin.

With other drugs

Metabolism of ethosuximide is inhibited by isoniazid, resulting in increased plasma concentration and risk of toxicity.

With alcohol/food

There are no known specific interactions between alcohol and ethosuximide, and there are no specific foods that must be excluded from diet when taking ethosuximide.

Special populations

Hepatic impairment
Use with caution.

Renal impairment
Use with caution.

Pregnancy

- The dose of ethosuximide should be monitored carefully during pregnancy and after delivery, and adjustments made on a clinical basis.
- Ethosuximide crosses the placenta and cases of birth defects have been reported. Therefore, the prescribing physician should weigh the benefits versus the risks of ethosuximide in treating or counselling epileptic women of childbearing age.
- Ethosuximide is excreted in breastmilk and the effects of ethosuximide on the nursing infant are unknown. Therefore, ethosuximide should be used in nursing mothers only if the benefits clearly outweigh the risks and breastfeeding is best avoided.

Behavioural and cognitive effects in patients with epilepsy

Adverse behavioural effects can be of clinical significance, and include the possible induction of anxiety, depression, confusion, irritability, aggression, hallucinations, and intermittent impairment of consciousness These episodes can occur following cessation of seizures and normalization of the electroencephalogram (EEG), and resolve with discontinuation of ethosuximide and seizure recurrence (alternative psychosis in the context of forced normalization). Among first-generation AEDs, ethosuximide is characterized by a relatively favourable cognitive profile, with low incidence of cognitive adverse effects.

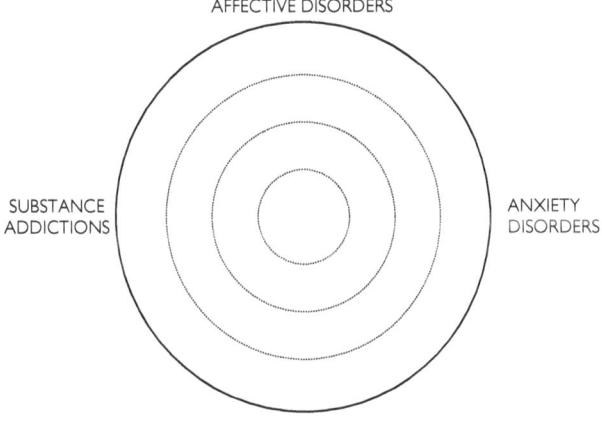

Fig. 5.3 Level of evidence supporting the psychiatric use of ethosuximide in patients with behavioural symptoms

Psychiatric use

Ethosuximide as adjunctive treatment of bipolar disorder was found to be ineffective in patients with acute mania. This AED has no approved indications or clinical uses in psychiatry (Fig. 5.3).

Overall rating

Ethosuximide is characterized by few antiepileptic indications, with an acceptable interaction profile in polytherapy. It has a good behavioural tolerability profile, but no psychiatric uses (Table 5.2).

Table 5.2 Overall rating of ethosuximide	
Antiepileptic indications	☺
Interactions in polytherapy	☺
Behavioural tolerability	☺☺
Psychiatric use	
Key: ☺☺☺ = very good; ☺☺ = good; ☺ = acceptable.	

CHAPTER 6

Gabapentin

Gabapentin is a second-generation antiepileptic drug (AED; Fig. 6.1) known under the proprietary brand name of Neurontin® (Pfizer, New York, NY) in the UK and USA (Fig. 6.2).

Preparation

Tablets
- Gabapentin 600 mg (100-tab pack).
- Gabapentin 800 mg (100-tab pack).

Capsules
- Gabapentin 100 mg (100-cap pack).
- Gabapentin 300 mg (100-cap pack).
- Gabapentin 400 mg (100-cap pack).

Oral solution
- Gabapentin 50 mg/mL (150 mL).

Generic formulation

MHRA/CHM advice to minimize risk when switching patients with epilepsy between different manufacturers' products (including generic products):

- *Category 3*: it is usually unnecessary to ensure that patients are maintained on a specific manufacturer's product unless there are specific concerns, such as patient anxiety and risk of confusion/dosing error.

Indications

Epilepsy: monotherapy or adjunctive therapy of focal seizures with or without secondary generalization.

56 • BEHAVIOURAL NEUROLOGY OF ANTIEPILEPTIC DRUGS

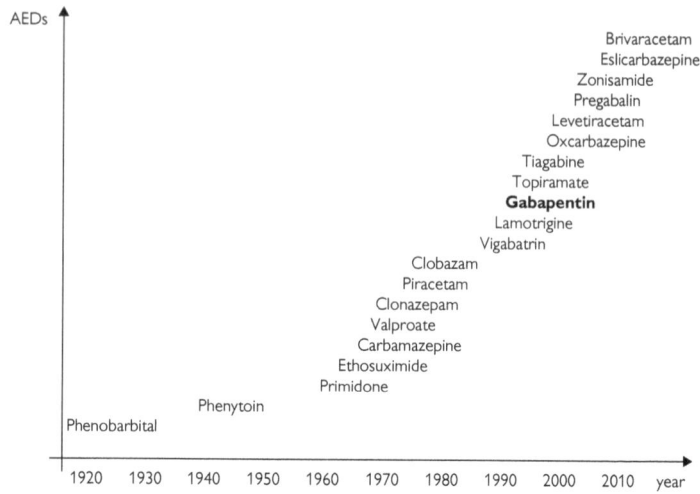

Fig. 6.1 Chronology of the clinical use of gabapentin

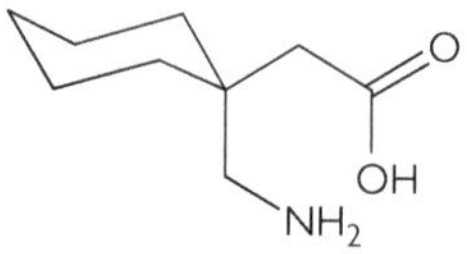

Fig. 6.2 Chemical structure of gabapentin

Recommendations summarized from NICE (2012)
- *Seizure types*: adjunctive (focal seizures), contraindicated (generalized tonic-clonic seizures generalized tonic-clonic seizures if there are absence or myoclonic seizures, or if juvenile myoclonic epilepsy is suspected, tonic/atonic seizures, absence seizures, myoclonic seizures).
- *Epilepsy types*: adjunctive (benign epilepsy with centrotemporal spikes, Panayiotopoulos syndrome, late-onset childhood occipital epilepsy), contraindicated (absence syndromes, juvenile myoclonic epilepsy, idiopathic generalized epilepsy, Dravet syndrome, Lennox–Gastaut syndrome)
  - *Psychiatry*— treatment of anxiety disorders (unlicensed); treatment of alcohol withdrawal symptoms (unlicensed).
  - *Neurology*—treatment of neuropathic pain and restless leg syndrome (unlicensed) and prophylaxis of migraine (unlicensed).

CHAPTER 6

Dose titration

Epilepsy

Monotherapy or adjunctive therapy

300 mg od for day 1300 mg bd for day 2300 mg td for day 3 (or 300 mg td for day 1), then increased by 300 mg every 2–3 days, divided into three doses; usual maintenance 900–3600 mg daily, divided into three doses (max. 4800 mg daily)

If gabapentin has to be discontinued, it is recommended this should be done gradually over a minimum of 1 week, independent of the indication.

Plasma levels monitoring

It is not necessary to monitor gabapentin plasma concentrations to optimize gabapentin therapy.

Cautions

- Patients with a history of psychotic illness.
- Patients with mixed seizures (including absences).
- Patients with diabetes mellitus.
- Elderly patients.

Adverse effects

Gabapentin can be associated with adverse effects at the level the nervous system and other systems (Table 6.1).

Interactions

With AEDs

Nil.

With other drugs

- Patients who require concomitant treatment with opioids should be carefully observed for signs of respiratory depression and/or sedation, and the dose of gabapentin or opioid should be reduced appropriately
- Co-administration of gabapentin with antacids containing aluminium and magnesium, reduces gabapentin bioavailability up to 24%, and it is therefore recommended that gabapentin be taken at the earliest 2 hours following antacid administration

Table 6.1 Estimated frequency of adverse effects of gabapentin

Very common (>1 in 10 patients on gabapentin)	
Nervous system • ataxia • dizziness • drowsiness	*Other systems* • fever
Common (>1 in 100 patients on gabapentin)	
Nervous system • Abnormal reflexes • abnormal thoughts • amnesia • anorexia • anxiety • confusion • convulsions • depression • emotional lability • headache • irritability • insomnia • movement disorders, tremor and twitching • nystagmus • paraesthesias • speech disorder • vertigo • visual disturbances	*Other systems* - Abdominal pain • acne • arthralgia • constipation and flatulence • cough • diarrhoea • dry mouth and throat • dyspepsia • dyspnoea • flu syndrome • gingivitis • hypertension • impotence • increased appetite and weight gain • leucopenia • malaise • myalgia • nausea and vomiting • oedema • pharyngitis and rhinitis • pruritus • rash • vasodilation
Uncommon (>1 in 1,000 patients on gabapentin)	
Nervous system • agitation • hypokinesia • mental impairment	*Other systems* • palpitations
Rare (>1 in 10,000 patients on gabapentin)	
Nervous system • loss of consciousness	*Other systems* • blood glucose fluctuations in patients with diabetes
Very rare (<1 in 10,000 patients on gabapentin)	
Nervous system	*Other systems*

With alcohol/food

There are no known specific interactions between alcohol and gabapentin and there are no specific foods that must be excluded from diet when taking gabapentin.

Special populations

Renal impairment

Reduce maintenance dose according to degree of reduction in creatinine clearance.

Pregnancy

- The dose of gabapentin should be monitored carefully during pregnancy and after birth, and adjustments made on a clinical basis.
- No definite conclusion can be made as to whether gabapentin is associated with an increased risk of congenital malformations when taken during pregnancy. Gabapentin should not be used during pregnancy unless the potential benefit to the mother clearly outweighs the potential risk to the foetus.
- Gabapentin is excreted in human milk. Because the effect on the breastfed infant is unknown, gabapentin should be used in breastfeeding mothers with caution and only if the benefits clearly outweigh the risks.

Behavioural and cognitive effects in patients with epilepsy

Gabapentin has a relatively favourable behavioural profile, although paradoxical hyperactivity, irritability and aggression have been occasionally reported, especially in patients with severe intellectual disabilities. The cognitive profile of gabapentin is equally favourable, as this AED has been associated with only minor cognitive difficulties (mainly in the attention domain).

Psychiatric use

Although gabapentin has no approved indications in psychiatry, it has shown efficacy in the treatment of anxiety disorders, especially social phobia. Other off-label uses include other anxiety disorders (panic disorder, post-traumatic stress disorder), alcohol dependence and withdrawal, behavioural and psychological symptoms of dementia, and aggression. Gabapentin has also been proposed to be useful in the maintenance treatment of bipolar disorder as adjunctive therapy (Fig. 6.3).

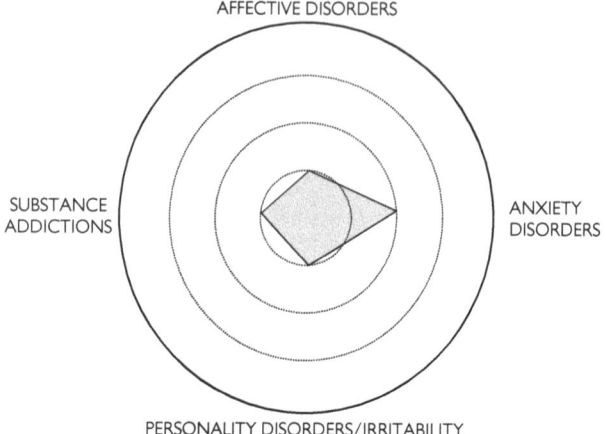

Fig. 6.3 Level of evidence supporting the psychiatric use of gabapentin in patients with behavioural symptoms

Overall rating

Gabapentin is characterized by few antiepileptic indications, with very good interaction profile in polytherapy; it has a good behavioural tolerability profile and a good range of psychiatric uses (Table 6.2).

Table 6.2 Overall rating of gabapentin	
Antiepileptic indications	☺
Interactions in polytherapy	☺ ☺ ☺
Behavioural tolerability	☺ ☺
Psychiatric use	☺ ☺
Key: ☺ ☺ ☺ = very good; ☺ ☺ = good; ☺ = acceptable.	

CHAPTER 7

Lamotrigine

Lamotrigine is a second-generation antiepileptic drug (AED; Fig. 7.1) known by the proprietary brand name of Lamictal® (GlaxoSmithKline, Brentford) in the UK and USA (Fig. 7.2).

Preparations

Tablets

- Lamotrigine 25 mg (56-tab pack).
- Lamotrigine 50 mg (56-tab pack).
- Lamotrigine 100 mg (56-tab pack).
- Lamotrigine 200 mg (56-tab pack).

Chewable/dispersible tablets

- Lamotrigine 2 mg (30-tab pack).
- Lamotrigine 5 mg (28-tab pack).
- Lamotrigine 25 mg (56-tab pack).
- Lamotrigine 100 mg (56-tab pack).

Generic formulation

MHRA/CHM advice to minimize risk when switching patients with epilepsy between different manufacturers' products (including generic products):

- *Category 2*: the need for continued supply of a particular manufacturer's product should be based on clinical judgment and consultation with the patient and/or carer taking into account factors such as seizure frequency and treatment history.

Indications

Epilepsy: monotherapy and adjunctive therapy of focal and generalized seizures.

62 • BEHAVIOURAL NEUROLOGY OF ANTIEPILEPTIC DRUGS

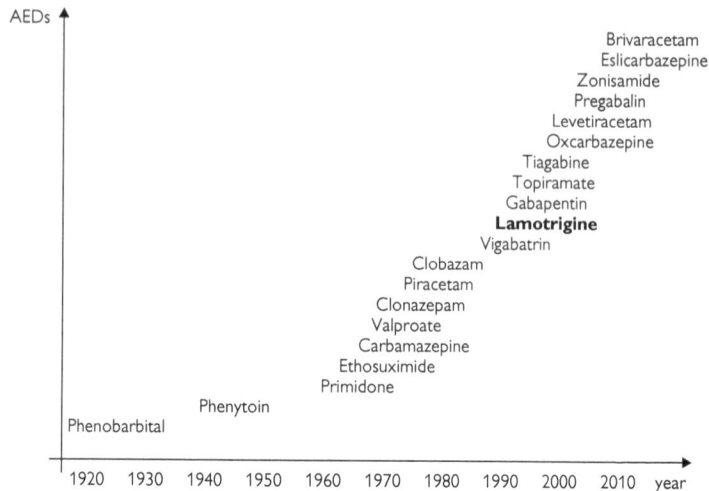

Fig. 7.1 Chronology of the clinical use of lamotrigine

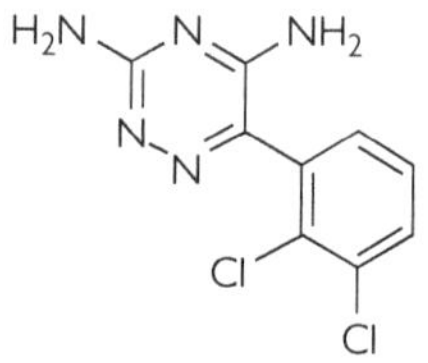

Fig. 7.2 Chemical structure of lamotrigine

Recommendations summarized from NICE (2012)

- *Seizure types*: first line (generalized tonic-clonic seizures, tonic/atonic seizures, absence seizures, focal seizures), adjunctive (generalized tonic-clonic seizures, absence seizures, focal seizures).
- *Epilepsy types*: first line (absence syndromes, juvenile myoclonic epilepsy, epilepsy with generalized tonic-clonic seizures only, idiopathic generalized epilepsy, benign epilepsy with centrotemporal spikes, Panayiotopoulos syndrome, late-onset childhood occipital epilepsy), adjunctive (absence syndromes, juvenile myoclonic epilepsy, epilepsy with generalized tonic-clonic seizures only, idiopathic generalized epilepsy, benign epilepsy with centrotemporal spikes, Panayiotopoulos syndrome, late-onset childhood occipital epilepsy, Lennox-Gastaut syndrome), contraindicated (Dravet syndrome)

Psychiatry: prevention of depressive episodes associated with bipolar disorder (not indicated for manic phase)

Dose titration

Epilepsy—monotherapy

25 mg od for 14 days, 50 mg od for 14 days, then increased to a maximum of 100 mg every 7–14 days; usual maintenance 100–200 mg daily, divided into 1–2 doses (max. 500 mg daily).

Epilepsy—adjunctive therapy (with valproate)

25 mg on alternate days for 14 days, 25 mg od for 14 days, then increased by a maximum of 50 mg every 7–14 days; usual maintenance 100–200 mg daily, divided into 1–2 doses (max. 500 mg daily).

Epilepsy—adjunctive therapy (with enzyme-inducing AED and without valproate)

50 mg od for 14 days, 50 mg bd for 14 days, then increased by a maximum of 100 mg every 7–14 days; usual maintenance 200–400 mg daily, divided into two doses (max. 700 mg daily).

Epilepsy—adjunctive therapy (without enzyme-inducing AED and without valproate)

25 mg od for 14 days, 50 mg od for 14 days, then increased by a maximum of 100 mg every 7–14 days; usual maintenance 100–200 mg daily, divided into 1 or 2 doses.

Bipolar disorder—monotherapy or adjunctive therapy (without enzyme-inducing AED and without valproate)

25 mg od for 14 days, 50 mg daily, divided into 1 or 2 doses for 14 days, 100 mg daily, divided into 1 or 2 doses for 7 days; usual maintenance 200 mg daily, divided into 1 or 2 doses (max. 400 mg daily).

Bipolar disorder—adjunctive therapy (with valproate)

25 mg on alternate days for 14 days, 25 mg od for 14 days, 50 mg daily, divided into 1 or 2 doses; usual maintenance 100 mg daily, divided into 1 or 2 doses (max. 200 mg daily).

Bipolar disorder—adjunctive therapy (with enzyme-inducing AED and without valproate)

50 mg od for 14 days, 50 mg bd for 14 days, 100 mg bd for 7 days; 150 mg bd for 7 days; usual maintenance 200 mg bd.

If stopping lamotrigine, patients with epilepsy need to reduce the dose gradually over about 2 weeks to minimize the risk of relapse. This does not apply to patients who take lamotrigine for bipolar disorder, although NICE (2015) recommend that it be reduced gradually over at least 4 weeks to minimize the risk of relapse.

Plasma levels monitoring

Although plasma levels can be measured, and a therapeutic range has been postulated (2.5–15 mg/L), there is only a loose relationship between serum concentration and clinical effectiveness/adverse effects. The routine measurement of plasma levels in clinical practice is therefore unnecessary, although it can sometimes be useful in guiding dosage adjustments in situations associated with changes in lamotrigine pharmacokinetics, such as pregnancy, puerperium, and polymedication.

Cautions

- Patients with a history of allergy or rash from other AEDs.
- Patients with Parkinson disease.
- Patients with myoclonic seizures.

Adverse effects

Lamotrigine can be associated with adverse effects at the level the nervous system and other systems (Table 7.1).

Interactions

With AEDs

- Plasma concentration of lamotrigine is increased by the glucuronidation inhibitor valproate (reduce lamotrigine dose to avoid increased risk of toxicity).
- Plasma concentration of lamotrigine is reduced by the glucuronidation inducers carbamazepine, phenytoin, phenobarbital and primidone.
- Lamotrigine can raise concentration of active metabolite of carbamazepine (conflicting evidence).

With other drugs

- Plasma concentration of lamotrigine is reduced by the glucuronidation inducers oestrogens, rifampicin, and ritonavir (consider increasing the dose of lamotrigine).
- Plasma concentration of lamotrigine is possibly increased by desogestrel.

Table 7.1 Estimated frequency of adverse effects of lamotrigine

Very common (>1 in 10 patients on lamotrigine)

Nervous system	Other systems
• headache	• skin rash

Common (>1 in 100 patients on lamotrigine)

Nervous system	Other systems
• aggression	• diarrhoea
• agitation	• dry mouth
• dizziness	• joint/muscle pain
• drowsiness	• nausea and vomiting
• insomnia	
• irritability	
• tiredness	
• tremor	

Uncommon (>1 in 1000 patients on lamotrigine)

Nervous system	Other systems
• ataxia	
• blurred vision	
• diplopia	

Rare (>1 in 10,000 patients on lamotrigine)

Nervous system	Other systems
• aseptic meningitis	• conjunctivitis
• nystagmus	• severe skin reaction (Stevens–Johnson syndrome)*

Very rare (<1 in 10,000 patients on lamotrigine)

Nervous system	Other systems
• confusion	• AED hypersensitivity syndrome (DRESS)
• hallucinations	• anaemia, leucopenia, thrombocytopenia or pancytopenia; aplastic anaemia
• tics, choeoatetosis or other involuntary movements	• disseminated intravascular coagulation
• worsening of Parkinson disease symptoms	• fever
• worsening of seizures	• liver problems
	• lupus erythematosus-like syndrome
	• oedema/lymphadenopathy
	• severe skin reaction (toxic epidermal necrolysis)

*Risk increased by concomitant use of valproate, high initial dose and rapid titration of lamotrigine.

With alcohol/food

There are no known specific interactions between alcohol and lamotrigine, and there are no specific foods that must be excluded from diet when taking lamotrigine.

Special populations

Hepatic impairment

- Halve dose in moderate impairment.
- Quarter dose in severe impairment.

Renal impairment

Reduce maintenance dose in significant impairment.

Pregnancy

- A large amount of data on pregnant women exposed to lamotrigine during the first trimester of pregnancy do not suggest a substantial increase in the teratogenity risk. However, if therapy with lamotrigine is considered necessary during pregnancy, the lowest possible therapeutic dose is recommended.
- Lamotrigine doses may need to be doubled during pregnancy, as its plasma clearance can greatly increase towards the end of pregnancy (dose adjustments made in pregnancy should be rapidly reversed in the few days after delivery).
- Should a woman on lamotrigine decide to breastfeed, the infant should be monitored for possible adverse effects, as lamotrigine can be excreted in considerable amounts in breastmilk. In combination with slow infantile elimination can result in plasma concentrations at which pharmacological effects occur

Behavioural and cognitive effects in patients with epilepsy

Lamotrigine is characterized by an overall positive psychotropic profile, especially in terms of antidepressant properties. There are mixed findings about its possible effects on anxiety symptoms. The main adverse behavioural effects include irritability, agitation, and aggression (especially in patients with learning disability). However, these are not very common. There is no evidence of a significantly increased risk of thought disorders or cognitive deficits (at least at commonly used therapeutic doses). Positive effects on cognitive functions seem to be associated with EEG changes, rather than enhanced cognition.

Psychiatric use

The use of lamotrigine for the treatment of behavioural symptoms emerged from the observation of mood improvement in patients taking this medication for partial epilepsy. The main use of lamotrigine in psychiatry settings is for the maintenance therapy of bipolar disorder (prevention of depressive episodes), for which there is an approved indication from both FDA and EMA. There is evidence of a modest benefit in acute bipolar depression and unipolar depression (especially in more severely depressed patients). Reassuring data show no increased risk for switch-over placebo, indicating that lamotrigine is a reasonable choice for the treatment of acute bipolar depression in patients already on mood stabilizers, including those who have demonstrated adverse effects, such as switching on commonly used antidepressants. Other off-label uses have been investigated with preliminary positive results in borderline personality disorder (anger, affective lability, impulsivity), whereas supportive evidence is limited for use in obsessive-compulsive disorder (augmentation therapy), post-traumatic stress disorder, schizophrenia, schizoaffective disorder, alcohol and opiate withdrawal, cocaine dependence, behavioural, and psychological symptoms of dementia (Fig. 7.3).

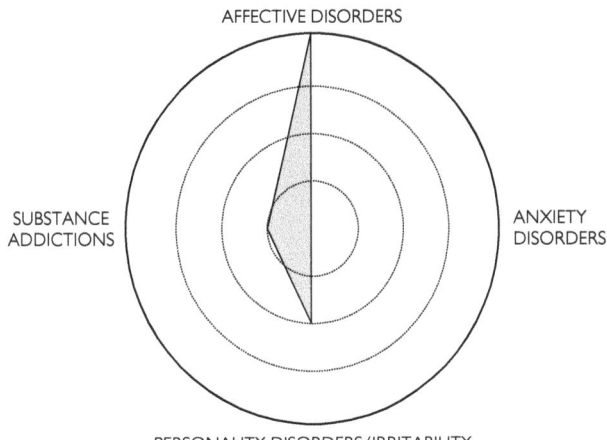

Fig. 7.3 Level of evidence supporting the psychiatric use of lamotrigine in patients with behavioural symptoms

Overall rating

Lamotrigine is characterized by a wide range of antiepileptic indications, with an acceptable interaction profile in polytherapy; it has a good behavioural tolerability profile and a wide range of psychiatric uses (Table 7.2).

Table 7.2 Overall rating of lamotrigine

Antiepileptic indications	☺ ☺ ☺
Interactions in polytherapy	☺
Behavioural tolerability	☺ ☺
Psychiatric use	☺ ☺ ☺

Key: ☺ ☺ ☺ = very good; ☺ ☺ = good; ☺ = acceptable.

CHAPTER 8

Levetiracetam, piracetam, and brivaracetam

Levetiracetam is a third-generation antiepileptic drug (AED; Fig. 8.1) known under the proprietary brand name of Keppra® (UCB Pharma, Slough) in the UK and USA (Fig. 8.2).

Preparations

Tablets

- Levetiracetam 250 mg (60-tab pack).
- Levetiracetam 500 mg (60-tab pack).
- Levetiracetam 750 mg (60-tab pack).
- Levetiracetam 1000 mg (60-tab pack).

Oral solution

Levetiracetam 100 mg/mL (300 mL).

Solution for infusion

Levetiracetam 100 mg/mL (50 mL).

Generic formulation

MHRA/CHM advice to minimize risk when switching patients with epilepsy between different manufacturers' products (including generic products):

- *Category 3*: it is usually unnecessary to ensure that patients are maintained on a specific manufacturer's product unless there are specific concerns, such as patient anxiety and risk of confusion/dosing error.

Indications

Epilepsy: monotherapy (not approved in USA) and adjunctive therapy of focal seizures with or without secondary generalization.

```
AEDs ▲
                                                              Brivaracetam
                                                              Eslicarbazepine
                                                              Zonisamide
                                                              Pregabalin
                                                              Levetiracetam
                                                              Oxcarbazepine
                                                           Tiagabine
                                                           Topiramate
                                                           Gabapentin
                                                           Lamotrigine
                                                         Vigabatrin
                                                Clobazam
                                                Piracetam
                                              Clonazepam
                                              Valproate
                                              Carbamazepine
                                             Ethosuximide
                                             Primidone
                             Phenytoin
         Phenobarbital
    ├─────┬─────┬─────┬─────┬─────┬─────┬─────┬─────┬─────┬─────►
    1920  1930  1940  1950  1960  1970  1980  1990  2000  2010  year
```

Fig. 8.1 Chronology of the clinical use of levetiracetam

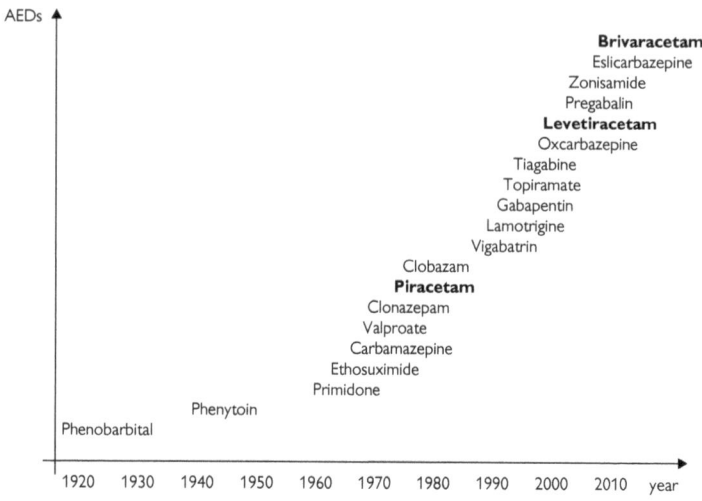

Fig. 8.2 Chemical structure of levetiracetam

Recommendations summarized from NICE (2012)

- *Seizure types*: first line (myoclonic seizures, focal seizures), adjunctive (generalized tonic-clonic seizures, myoclonic seizures, focal seizures), on referral to tertiary care (absence seizures).
- *Epilepsy types*: first line (juvenile myoclonic epilepsy, benign epilepsy with centrotemporal spikes, Panayiotopoulos syndrome, late-onset childhood occipital epilepsy), adjunctive (juvenile myoclonic epilepsy, epilepsy with generalized tonic-clonic seizures only, idiopathic generalized epilepsy, benign epilepsy with centrotemporal spikes, Panayiotopoulos syndrome, late-onset childhood occipital epilepsy).

Dose titration

Epilepsy—monotherapy

250 mg od for 7–14 days, 250 mg bd for 14 days, then increased by 250 mg bd every 14 days (max. maintenance dose 1500 mg bd).

Epilepsy—adjunctive therapy

250 mg bd for 14 days, then increased by 500 mg bd every 14–28 days (max. maintenance dose 1500 mg bd).

If levetiracetam has to be discontinued, it is recommended to withdraw it gradually (e.g. in patients weighing more than 50 kg: 500 mg decreases bd every 14–28 days).

Plasma levels monitoring

Due to its complete and linear absorption, plasma levels can be predicted from the oral dose of levetiracetam and, therefore, there is no need for plasma level monitoring of levetiracetam.

Cautions

Nil.

Adverse effects

Levetiracetam can be associated with adverse effects at the level of the nervous system and other systems (Table 8.1).

Interactions

With AEDs

Nil

With other drugs

- Concomitant administration of levetiracetam and methotrexate has been reported to decrease methotrexate clearance, resulting in increased/prolonged blood methotrexate concentration to potentially toxic levels.
- There have been isolated reports of decreased levetiracetam efficacy when the osmotic laxative macrogol has been concomitantly administered with levetiracetam. Therefore, macrogol should not be taken orally for 1 hour before or after taking levetiracetam.

Table 8.1 Estimated frequency of adverse effects of levetiracetam.

Very common (>1 in 10 patients on levetiracetam)

Nervous system	Other systems
• drowsiness • headache	• nasopharingitis

Common (>1 in 100 patients on levetiracetam)

nervous system	Other systems
• aggression • anorexia • anxiety • ataxia • convulsions • depression • dizziness • insomnia • irritability • tiredness • tremor • vertigo	• abdominal pain • cough • diarrhoea • dysepsia • malaise • nausea and vomiting

Uncommon (>1 in 1000 patients on levetiracetam)

Nervous system	Other systems
• agitation • amnesia • blurred vision • confusion • diplopia • impaired attention • paraesthesias • psychosis • suicidal ideation	• alopecia • eczema • leucopenia • myalgia • pruritus • thrombocytopenia • weight changes

Rare (>1 in 10,000 patients on levetiracetam)

Nervous system	Other systems
• choeoatetosis or other involuntary movements	• agranulocytosis • AED hypersensitivity syndrome (DRESS) • erythema multiforme • hyponatremia • liver problems • neutropenia • pancreatitis • pancytopenia • severe skin reactions (Stevens–Johnson syndrome, toxic epidermal necrolysis)

Very rare (<1 in 10,000 patients on levetiracetam)

Nervous system	Other systems

With alcohol/food
There are no known specific interactions between alcohol and levetiracetam, and there are no specific foods that must be excluded from diet when taking levetiracetam.

Special populations

Hepatic impairment
Halve dose in severe impairment with significant reduction in creatinine clearance

Renal impairment
Reduce maintenance dose according to degree of reduction in creatinine clearance

Pregnancy
- Post-marketing data from several prospective pregnancy registries of women exposed to levetiracetam monotherapy during the first trimester of pregnancy do not suggest a substantial increase in the risk for major congenital malformations, although a teratogenic risk cannot be completely excluded (especially in polytherapy with AEDs). Levetiracetam is not recommended during pregnancy or in women of childbearing age not using contraception unless clinically necessary.
- Decrease in levetiracetam plasma concentrations has been observed during pregnancy (especially during the third trimester), suggesting that appropriate clinical management of pregnant women treated with levetiracetam should be ensured
- Levetiracetam is excreted in human breastmilk and, therefore, breastfeeding is not recommended. However, if levetiracetam treatment is needed during breastfeeding, the benefit/risk of the treatment should be weighed up.

Behavioural and cognitive effects in patients with epilepsy
Behavioural adverse event are often reported by patients with epilepsy taking levetiracetam. The most relevant ones are irritability and emotional lability. Marked behavioural changes with psychotic symptoms and episodes of severe aggression have occasionally been reported. On the contrary, levetiracetam is one of the safest AEDs in terms of interference with cognitive processes, despite occasional reports of decreased cognition.

Psychiatric use
Despite its widespread use in epilepsy, levetiracetam does not have approved indications in psychiatry. Initial reports suggesting a possible role for levetiracetam

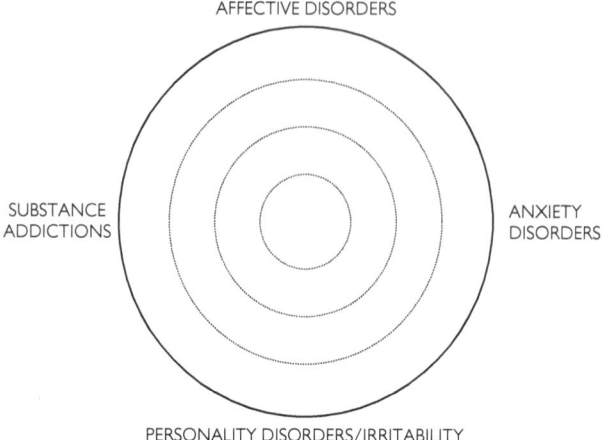

Fig. 8.3 Level of evidence supporting the psychiatric use of levetiracetam in patients with behavioural symptoms

in the treatment of bipolar depression and anxiety disorders have not been confirmed by the findings of controlled trials. Evidence for the possible usefulness of levetiracetam for the treatment of patients with Tourette syndrome is equally inconsistent (Fig. 8.3).

Overall rating

Levetiracetam is characterized by a wide range of antiepileptic indications, with a very good interaction profile in polytherapy. It has an acceptable behavioural tolerability profile and limited potential for psychiatric uses (Table 8.2).

Table 8.2 Overall rating of levetiracetam

Antiepileptic indications	☺ ☺ ☺
Interactions in polytherapy	☺ ☺ ☺
Behavioural tolerability	☺
Psychiatric use	☺

Key: ☺ ☺ ☺ = very good; ☺ ☺ = good; ☺ = acceptable.

Piracetam

Found commercially under the name Nootropil® (UCB Pharma, Slough, UK) Piracetam is available in tablet form (800 mg) and as oral solution (333.3 mg/mL). Piracetam is initially prescribed at a dose of 7.2 g daily, divided into 2 or 3 doses, and can be gradually increased in steps of 4.8 g daily every 3–4 days up to a maximum dose of 20 g daily (subsequently, attempts should be made to reduce the dose of concurrent therapy). Piracetam is a nootropic agent with an indication as adjunctive treatment for myoclonus of cortical origin, as well as tardive dyskinesia. However, piracetam is not approved by the FDA for any medical use in the USA. Piracetam should not be prescribed in patients with Huntington disease, those with serious kidney problems, or patients who have experienced a brain haemorrhage. Bleeding problems are a further caution to be taken into account. Most common adverse effects are hyperkinesia, irritability, and weight gain; less commonly, patients can report asthenia, depression, and drowsiness. Although there is little evidence for piracetam's efficacy in terms of long-term benefits for the treatment of mild cognitive impairments, recent studies showed that it is effective in the treatment of cognitive disorders of cerebrovascular and traumatic origins. With regard to piracetam's behavioural profile, its beneficial effects on lowering depression and anxiety appear to be higher than its positive effects on memory.

Brivaracetam

Brivaracetam is known under the proprietary name of Briviact® (UCB Pharma, Slough) in the UK and USA.

Brivaracetam is available in different pharmaceutical forms (10-25-50-75-100 mg film-coated tablets and 10 mg/mL oral solution). Brivaracetam is initially prescribed at the dose of 50–100 mg daily, divided into two doses. Based on individual patient response and tolerability, the dose may be adjusted within the dose range of 50–200 mg daily. Brivaracetam is recommended as an adjunctive AED treatment for partial-onset seizures with or without secondary generalization. Brivaracetam exhibits greater antiepileptic properties than levetiracetam in animal models, but with a somewhat smaller (although still high) therapeutic range. Moreover, brivaracetam requires no up-titration to reach therapeutic doses and there is no recommendation for specific monitoring. Exposure to brivaracetam is increased in patients with chronic liver disease. A starting dose of 50 mg daily should be considered and a maximum daily dose of 150 mg administered, divided into two doses, is recommended for all stages of hepatic impairment. If patients missed one dose or more, it is recommended that they take a single dose as soon as they remember and take the following dose at the usual morning or evening time, in order to avoid the brivaracetam plasma concentration falling below the efficacy level and prevent breakthrough seizures from occurring. If brivaracetam has to be discontinued, it is recommended to withdraw it gradually by 50 mg daily on a weekly basis. After 1 week of treatment at 50 mg daily, a final week of treatment at the dose of 20 mg daily is recommended. There is a limited amount of data from the use of brivaracetam in pregnant women. As the potential risk for humans is unknown, brivaracetam should not be used during pregnancy unless the benefit to the mother clearly outweighs the potential risk to the foetus. Likewise, it is unknown whether brivaracetam is excreted in human breastmilk and a decision should be made whether to discontinue breastfeeding or to discontinue brivaracetam, taking into account the benefit of the medicinal product to the mother. The most frequently reported adverse reactions associated with brivaracetam treatment are somnolence and dizziness (both somnolence and fatigue are reported with a higher incidence with increasing dose). Preliminary meta-analytic data comparing the incidence of behavioural problems in brivaracetam and levetiracetam trials (used as adjunctive therapy in adults with uncontrolled partial-onset epilepsy) showed that the incidence of non-psychotic behavioural treatment emergent adverse effects was considerably lower with brivaracetam treatment (6.8%) compared with levetiracetam (10.9%), whereas the incidences in placebo arms were similar (4.2 and 4.8%, respectively). The placebo-adjusted incidence rates were 2.6% for brivaracetam and 6.1% for levetiracetam, resulting in a brivaracetam/levetiracetam Odds Ratio of 0.68. Brivaracetam has a low interaction potential, although it is not recommended for use with concomitant levetiracetam.

CHAPTER 9

Phenobarbital and primidone

Phenobarbital and primidone are non-proprietary first-generation antiepileptic drugs (AEDs; Figs 9.1–9.3).

Preparations

Phenobarbital

Tablets

- Phenobarbital 15 mg (28-tab pack).
- Phenobarbital 30 mg (28-tab pack).
- Phenobarbital 60 mg (28-tab pack).

Oral solution

Phenobarbital 3 mg/mL (500 mL).

Primidone

Tablets

- Primidone 50 mg (100-tab pack).
- Primidone 250 mg (100-tab pack).

Generic formulation

MHRA/CHM advice is to minimize risk when switching patients with epilepsy between different manufacturers' products (including generic products):

- *Category 1*: doctors are advised to ensure that their patients are maintained on a specific manufacturer's product.

Indications

Epilepsy: monotherapy and adjunctive therapy of all seizures apart from focal seizures.

78 • BEHAVIOURAL NEUROLOGY OF ANTIEPILEPTIC DRUGS

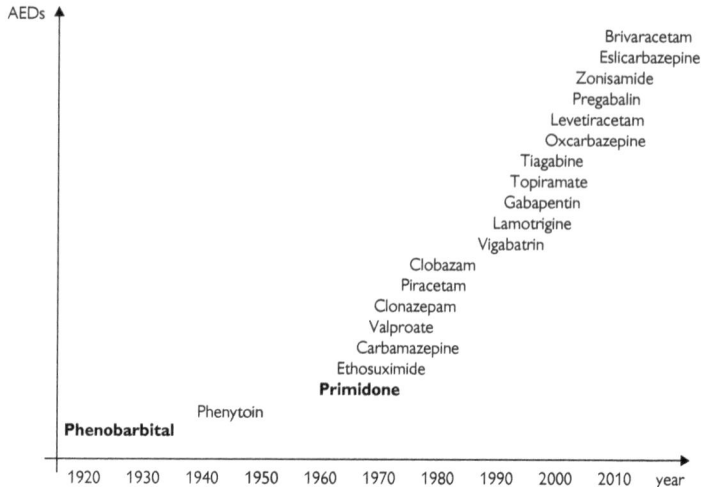

Fig. 9.1 Chronology of the clinical use of phenobarbital and primidone

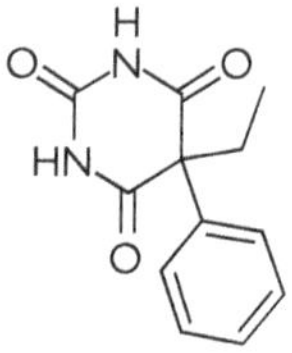

Fig. 9.2 Chemical structure of phenobarbital

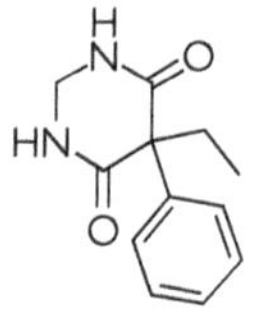

Fig. 9.3 Chemical structure of primidone

Phenobarbital

Recommendations summarized from NICE (2012)
- *Seizure types*: on referral to tertiary care (focal seizures).
- *Epilepsy types*: on referral to tertiary care (idiopathic generalized epilepsy, benign epilepsy with centrotemporal spikes, Panayiotopoulos syndrome, late-onset childhood occipital epilepsy).

Primidone

Neurology: treatment of essential tremor.

Dose titration

Phenobarbital
Epilepsy: 60–180 mg nocte.

Primidone
Epilepsy—monotherapy: 125 mg nocte, increased by 125 mg every 3 days to 500 mg daily, divided into two doses, then increased by 250 mg every 3 days; usual maintenance 75–1500 mg daily, divided into two doses.

Plasma levels monitoring

Plasma phenobarbital concentration for optimum response is 15–40 mg/L; however, monitoring the plasma concentration is less useful than with other drugs because tolerance occurs. For primidone, it is possible to monitor plasma concentrations of derived phenobarbital as required.

Cautions

- Patients with a history of alcohol or drug abuse.
- Elderly or debilitated patients.
- Patients with acute porphyrias.
- Patients with respiratory depression.

Adverse effects

Phenobarbital can be associated with adverse effects at the level the nervous system and other systems (Table 9.1).

Table 9.1 Estimated frequency of adverse effects of phenobarbital

Very common or common (>1 in 10 or >1 in 100 patients on phenobarbital)	
Nervous system	Other systems
• amnesia	• agranulocytosis
• ataxia	• allergic skin reactions
• behavioural disturbances	• anaemia
• depression	• cholestasis
• drowsiness	• hepatitis
• hallucinations	• hypotension
• impaired cognition	• osteomalacia
• irritability	• respiratory depression
• lethargy	• thrombocytopenia
• nystagmus	
• paradoxical excitement and hyperactivity (especially in the elderly)	
Uncommon (>1 in 1000 patients on phenobarbital)	
Nervous system	Other systems
Rare (>1 in 10,000 patients on phenobarbital)	
Nervous system	Other systems
• Psychosis	• arthralgia
	• systemic lupus erythematosus
Very rare (<1 in 10,000 patients on phenobarbital)	
Nervous system	Other systems
	• AED hypersensitivity syndrome (DRESS)
	• severe skin reaction (Stevens–Johnson syndrome, toxic epidermal necrolysis)
	• suicidal ideation

Primidone can be associated with adverse effects at the level the nervous system and other systems (Table 9.2).

Interactions

With AEDs

- Both primidone and its major metabolite phenobarbital are metabolized by, and also induce, liver enzyme activity (especially the CYP 450 3A4 enzyme system). There are a number of interactions which are potentially clinically significant.

Table 9.2 Estimated frequency of adverse effects of primidone

Very common or common (>1 in 10 or >1 in 100 patients on primidone)

Nervous system	Other systems
• amnesia	• agranulocytosis
• ataxia	• allergic skin reactions
• behavioural disturbances	• anaemia
• depression	• cholestasis
• drowsiness	• hepatitis
• hallucinations	• hypotension
• impaired cognition	• nausea
• irritability	• osteomalacia
• lethargy	• respiratory depression
• nystagmus	• thrombocytopenia
• paradoxical excitement and hyperactivity (especially in the elderly)	
• visual disturbances	

Uncommon (>1 in 1000 patients on primidone)

Nervous system	Other systems
• dizziness	• vomiting
• headache	

Rare (>1 in 10,000 patients on primidone)

Nervous system	Other systems
• psychosis	• arthralgia systemic lupus erythematosus

Very rare (<1 in 10,000 patients on primidone)

Nervous system	Other systems
	• AED hypersensitivity syndrome (DRESS)
	• severe skin reaction (Stevens–Johnson syndrome, toxic epidermal necrolysis)
	• suicidal ideation

- Phenobarbital and primidone plasma concentrations are increased by oxcarbazepine, phenytoin and valproate.
- Vigabatrin possibly decreases phenobarbital and primidone plasma concentrations.
- Phenobarbital and primidone therapy may also lead to altered pharmacokinetics in concomitantly administered AEDs, whose metabolism may be increased, and lead to lowered plasma levels and/or a shorter half-life: carbamazepine, ethosuximide, lamotrigine, oxcarbazepine, phenytoin, valproate, tiagabine, topiramate, zonisamide.

With other drugs

- Agents which inhibit the CYP 450 3A4 enzyme system, such as chloramphenicol, nelfinavir, and metronidazole may result in increased plasma levels of concomitantly administered primidone and its metabolite phenobarbital.
- In addition, St John's wort induces the CYP450 enzyme system and may result in a reduction of plasma levels of concomitantly administered primidone and of its metabolite phenobarbital.
- Phenobarbital and primidone therapy may also lead to altered pharmacokinetics in concomitantly administered drugs, whose metabolism may be increased, and lead to lowered plasma levels and/or a shorter half-life. These drugs include androgens, beta-antagonists, ciclosporin, clozapine, chloramphenicol, corticosteroids/glucocorticosteroids, cyclophosphamide, dicoumarins, digitoxin, doxycycline, etoposide, granisetron, losartan, methadone, metronidazole, mianserin, montelukast, nelfinavir, nimodipine, oral contraceptives, quinidine, rocuronium, theophyllines, tricyclic antidepressants, vecuronium, and warfarin.
- The central nervous system (CNS) depressant effect of phenobarbital and primidone is additive to those of other CNS depressants such as opiates.

With alcohol/food

Concurrent administration with alcohol may lead to an additive CNS depressant effect and there are no specific foods that must be excluded from diet when taking phenobarbital or primidone.

Special populations

Hepatic impairment

Reduce dose as it may precipitate coma (avoid in severe impairment).

Renal impairment

Use with caution.

Pregnancy

- Phenobarbital and primidone therapy in pregnant women with epilepsy present a risk to the foetus in terms of major and minor congenital defects, such as congenital craniofacial, heart, and digital abnormalities, as well as cleft lip and palate.
- In case of treatment during pregnancy, the dose of phenobarbital and primidone should be monitored carefully and adjustments made on a clinical basis.

- Phenobarbital and primidone readily cross the placenta following oral administration and are distributed throughout foetal tissue, the highest concentrations being found in the placenta, foetal liver and brain. Adverse effects on neurobehavioural development and withdrawal symptoms have been reported in the newly born whose mothers have received phenobarbital or primidone during late pregnancy
- Phenobarbital and primidone are excreted into breastmilk and there is a small risk of neonatal sedation. During breastfeeding, the baby should be monitored for sedation, although breastfeeding is not advisable.

Behavioural and cognitive effects in patients with epilepsy

Patients taking phenobarbital have been shown to have a high prevalence of major depressive disorder and suicidal ideation. A long history of exposure to barbiturates may carry the greatest risk of depression, particularly in patients taking polytherapy and patients with a personal or family history of affective disorders. Similarly to benzodiazepines, barbiturates can also induce a paradoxycal syndrome characterized by insomnia, hyperactivity, impulsiveness and aggressiveness (especially in patients with learning disability). Barbiturates are more frequently associated with adverse cognitive side effects than most other AEDs. The spectrum of cognitive problems reported by patients with epilepsy taking phenobarbital encompasses attention, memory, and language.

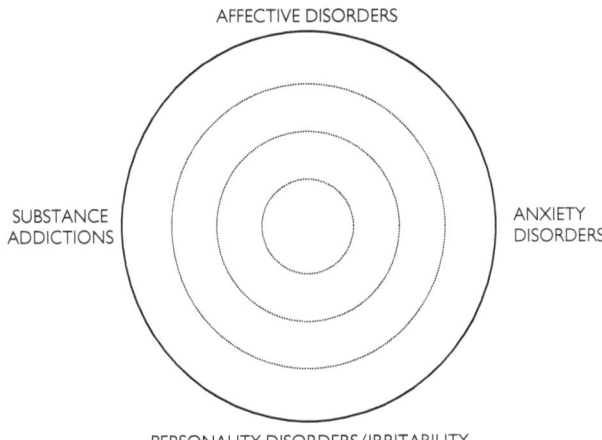

Fig. 9.4 Level of evidence supporting the psychiatric use of phenobarbital and primidone in patients with behavioural symptoms

Psychiatric use

Barbiturates have no approved indications in psychiatry. Off-label uses have previously included sedative-hypnotic withdrawal and alcohol-withdrawal (as alternative to benzodiazepines) (Fig. 9.4).

Overall rating

Phenobarbital and primidone are characterized by a restricted range of antiepileptic indications, with an acceptable interaction profile in polytherapy. These drugs have an acceptable behavioural tolerability profile, but no clinical uses in psychiatry (Table 9.3).

Table 9.3 Overall rating of phenobarbital and primidone	
Antiepileptic indications	☺
Interactions in polytherapy	☺
Behavioural tolerability	☺
Psychiatric use	
Key: ☺☺☺ = very good; ☺☺ = good; ☺ = acceptable.	

CHAPTER 10

Phenytoin

Phenytoin is a first-generation antiepileptic drug (AED; Fig. 10.1) known with the proprietary brand name of Epanutin® (Pfizer, Tadworth) in the UK and Dilantin® (Pfizer, New York, NY) in the USA (Fig. 10.2).

Preparations

Tablets
Phenytoin 100 mg (28-tab pack).

Capsules
- Phenytoin 25 mg (28-cap pack).
- Phenytoin 50 mg (28-cap pack).
- Phenytoin 100 mg (84-cap pack).
- Phenytoin 300 mg (28-cap pack).

Oral suspension
Phenytoin 6 mg/mL (500 mL).

Generic formulation

MHRA/CHM advice to minimize risk when switching patients with epilepsy between different manufacturers' products (incl. generic products):

- *Category 1*: doctors are advised to ensure that their patients are maintained on a specific manufacturer's product.

```
AEDs
                                                      Brivaracetam
                                                      Eslicarbazepine
                                                      Zonisamide
                                                      Pregabalin
                                                      Levetiracetam
                                                      Oxcarbazepine
                                                   Tiagabine
                                                   Topiramate
                                                   Gabapentin
                                                   Lamotrigine
                                                Vigabatrin
                                       Clobazam
                                       Piracetam
                                     Clonazepam
                                     Valproate
                                     Carbamazepine
                                    Ethosuximide
                                    Primidone
                        Phenytoin
        Phenobarbital
        1920  1930  1940  1950  1960  1970  1980  1990  2000  2010  year
```

Fig. 10.1 Chronology of the clinical use of phenytoin

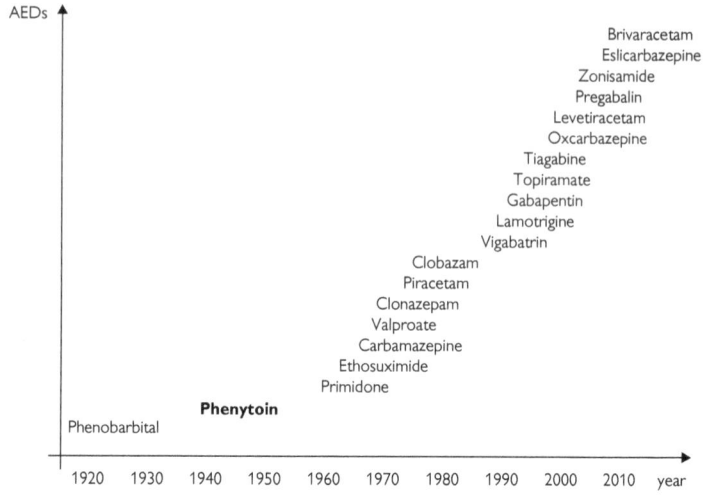

Fig. 10.2 Chemical structure of phenytoin

Indications

Epilepsy

Monotherapy and adjunctive therapy of focal and generalized tonic-clonic seizures.

Recommendations summarized from NICE (2012)

- *Seizure types*: on referral to tertiary care (focal seizures), contraindicated (generalized tonic-clonic seizures if there are absence or myoclonic seizures or if juvenile myoclonic epilepsy is suspected, absence seizures, myoclonic seizures).
- *Epilepsy types*: on referral to tertiary care (benign epilepsy with centrotemporal spikes, Panayiotopoulos syndrome, late-onset childhood occipital epilepsy), contraindicated (absence syndromes, juvenile myoclonic epilepsy, idiopathic generalized epilepsy, Dravet syndrome).

Dose titration

Epilepsy

150–300 mg od or divided into two doses, then increased to 200–500 mg daily (dose to be increased gradually as necessary, with plasma phenytoin concentration monitoring).

Plasma levels monitoring

Phenytoin has a narrow therapeutic index and the relationship between dose and plasma. Phenytoin concentration is non-linear: small dosage increases in some patients may produce large increases in plasma concentration with acute toxic adverse effects. Similarly, a few missed doses or a small change in phenytoin absorption may result in a marked change in plasma phenytoin concentration. Monitoring of plasma phenytoin concentration improves dosage adjustments. The usual total plasma phenytoin concentration for optimum response is 10–20 mg/L (careful interpretation of total plasma phenytoin concentration is necessary in pregnancy, the elderly, and certain disease states where protein binding may be reduced and it may be more appropriate to measure free plasma phenytoin concentration).

Cautions

Patients with acute porphyrias (contraindication).

Adverse effects

See Table 10.1.

Interactions

With AEDs

- Phenytoin is extensively bound to serum plasma proteins and is prone to competitive displacement. Phenytoin is metabolized by hepatic enzymes (cytochrome P450 CYP2C9 and CYP2C19) and is particularly susceptible to inhibitory drug interactions because it is subject to saturable metabolism.
- Several AEDs, including eslicarbazepine, oxcarbazepine, topiramate, and valproate, potentially increase phenytoin serum levels.
- Vigabatrin may decrease phenytoin plasma levels.
- Carbamazepine, phenobarbital, and valproate may either increase or decrease phenytoin serum levels.

Table 10.1 Estimated frequency of adverse effects of phenytoin

Very common or common (>1 in 10 or >1 in 100 patients on phenytoin)

Nervous system	Other systems
• dizziness	• acne
• drowsiness	• anorexia
• headache	• coarsening of facial appearance
• insomnia	• constipation
• irritability	• gingival hypertrophy
• paraesthesias	• hirsutism
• tremor	• nausea and vomiting
	• rash

Uncommon (>1 in 1000 patients on phenytoin)

Nervous system	Other systems

Rare (>1 in 10,000 patients on phenytoin)

Nervous system	Other systems
• dyskinesias	• blood disorders (anaemia, leucopenia, thrombocytopenia)
• peripheral neuropathy	• hepatotoxicity
	• lupus erythematosus
	• lymphadenopathy
	• osteomalacia
	• polyarteritis nodosa
	• severe skin reactions (Stevens–Johnson syndrome, toxic epidermal necrolysis)*

Very rare (<1 in 10,000 patients on phenytoin)

Nervous system	Other systems

*Before deciding to initiate treatment, patients of Han Chinese and Thai origin should, whenever possible, be screened for HLA-B*1502, as this allele strongly predicts the risk of severe phenytoin-associated Stevens–Johnson syndrome.

- Phenytoin is a potent inducer of hepatic drug-metabolizing enzymes and may reduce the levels of drugs metabolized by these enzymes.
- Phenytoin may alter serum levels and/or effects of carbamazepine, lamotrigine, phenobarbital, and valproate.

With other drugs

- Phenytoin serum levels are potentially increased by analgesic/anti-inflammatory agents (such as azapropazone, phenylbutazone, salicylates), anaesthetics (halothane), antibacterial agents (such as chloramphenicol, erythromycin, isoniazid, sulfadiazine, sulfamethizole, sulfamethoxazole-trimethoprim, sulfaphenazole, sulfisoxazole, sulfonamides), antifungal agents (such as amphotericin, fluconazole, itraconazole, ketoconazole, miconazole, voriconazole), antineoplastic agents (such as capecitabine, fluorouracil), psychotropic agents (such as chlordiazepoxide, diazepam, disulfiram, fluoxetine, fluvoxamine, methylphenidate, sertraline, trazodone, viloxazine), cardiovascular agents (such as amiodarone, dicoumarol, diltiazem, nifedipine, ticlopidine), H2-antagonists (such as cimetidine), HMG-CoA reductase inhibitors (such as fluvastatin), hormones (such as oestrogens), immunosuppressant drugs (such as tacrolimus), oral hypoglycaemic agents (such as tolbutamide), proton pump inhibitors (such as omeprazole).

• Phenytoin plasma levels may be decreased by antibacterial agents (such as ciprofloxacin, rifampicin), antineoplastic agents (such as bleomycin, carboplatin, cisplatin, doxorubicin, methotrexate), antiulcer agents (such as sucralfate), antiretrovirals (such as fosamprenavir, nelfinavir, ritonavir), bronchodilators (such as theophylline), cardiovascular agents (such as reserpine), folic acid, hyperglycaemic agents (such as diazoxide), St John's wort (*Hypericum perforatum*).

• Phenytoin serum levels may be either increased or decreased by antibacterial agents (such as ciprofloxacin), antineoplastic agents, and psychotropic agents (such as chlordiazepoxide, diazepam, and phenothiazines).

• Phenytoin may alter serum levels and/or effects of the following drugs: antibacterial agents (such as doxycycline, rifampicin, tetracycline), antifungal agents (such as azoles, posaconazole, voriconazole), antihelminthics (such as albendazole, praziquantel), antineoplastic agents (such as teniposide), antiretrovirals (such as delavirdine, efavirenz, fosamprenavir, indinavir, lopinavir/ritonavir, nelfinavir, ritonavir, saquinavir), bronchodilators (such as theophylline), cardiovascular agents (such as digitoxin, digoxin, mexiletine, nicardipine, nimodipine, nisoldipine, quinidine, verapamil), coumarin anticoagulants (such as warfarin), ciclosporin, diuretics (such as furosemide), HMG-CoA reductase inhibitors (such as atorvastatin, fluvastatin, simvastatin), hormones (such as oestrogens, oral contraceptives), hyperglycaemic agents (such as diazoxide), immunosuppressant drugs, neuromuscular blocking agents (such as alcuronium, cisatracurium, pancuronium, rocuronium, vecuronium), opioid analgesics (such as methadone), oral hypoglycaemic agents (such as chlorpropamide, glyburide, tolbutamide), psychotropic agents (such as clozapine, paroxetine, quetiapine, sertraline), vitamin D.

With alcohol/food

Acute alcohol intake may increase phenytoin serum levels while chronic alcoholism may decrease serum levels. There are no specific foods that must be excluded from diet when taking phenytoin (phenytoin doses should be taken preferably with or after food).

Special populations

Hepatic impairment
Reduce dose to avoid toxicity.

Renal impairment
Nil.

Pregnancy
- Phenytoin may produce congenital abnormalities in the offspring of a small number of epileptic patients. Therefore, phenytoin should only be used during pregnancy, especially early pregnancy, if in the judgement of the physician the potential benefits clearly outweigh the risk.
- In addition to the reports of increased incidence of congenital malformations, such as cleft lip/palate and heart malformations in children of women receiving phenytoin, there have been reports of a foetal hydantoin syndrome, consisting of prenatal growth deficiency, micro-encephaly, and mental deficiency in children born to mothers who have received phenytoin. There have been isolated reports of malignancies, including neuroblastoma, in children whose mothers received phenytoin during pregnancy.
- An increase in seizure frequency during pregnancy occurs in a proportion of patients, possibly due to altered phenytoin absorption or metabolism. Therefore, periodic measurement of serum phenytoin levels is particularly valuable in the management of a pregnant patient with epilepsy as a guide to an appropriate adjustment of dosage; however, postpartum restoration of the original dosage will probably be indicated.
- Breast-feeding is not recommended for women taking phenytoin because phenytoin appears to be secreted in low concentrations in human milk.

Behavioural and cognitive effects in patients with epilepsy

Phenytoin has an overall favourable behavioural profile, although it has been occasionally associated with negative effects on mood and psychotic symptoms (especially at higher doses). The cognitive profile is more problematic, especially in the attention and memory domains. Cognitive adverse effects associated with phenytoin are often dose-dependent and may be particularly obvious in visually guided motor functions.

Psychiatric use

Phenytoin has no approved indications in psychiatry, although the results of small randomized studies have shown that it may be useful in the maintenance treatment of bipolar disorder, major depressive disorder, and impulsive aggression (Fig. 10.3).

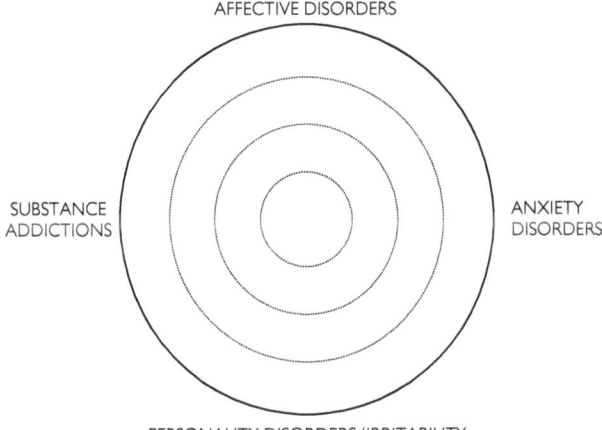

Fig. 10.3 Level of evidence supporting the psychiatric use of phenytoin in patients with behavioural symptoms

Overall rating

Phenytoin is characterized by a good range of antiepileptic indications, with an acceptable interaction profile in polytherapy; it has a good behavioural tolerability profile and a restricted range of psychiatric uses (Table 10.2).

Table 10.2 Overall rating of phenytoin	
Antiepileptic indications	☺ ☺
Interactions in polytherapy	☺
Behavioural tolerability	☺ ☺
Psychiatric use	☺
Key: ☺ ☺ ☺ = very good; ☺ ☺ = good; ☺ = acceptable.	

CHAPTER 11

Pregabalin

Pregabalin is a second-generation antiepileptic drug (AED; (Fig. 11.1) known with the proprietary brand name of Lyrica® (Pfizer, Tadworth) in the UK and USA (Pfizer, New York, NY; Fig. 11.2).

Preparations

Capsules
- Pregabalin 25 mg (56-cap pack).
- Pregabalin 50 mg (84-cap pack).
- Pregabalin 75 mg (56-cap pack).
- Pregabalin 100 mg (84-cap pack).
- Pregabalin 150 mg (56-cap pack).
- Pregabalin 200 mg (84-cap pack).
- Pregabalin 225 mg (56-cap pack).
- Pregabalin 300 mg (56-cap pack).

Oral solution
Pregabalin 20 mg/1 mL (473 mL).

Generic formulation

MHRA/CHM advice to minimize risk when switching patients with epilepsy between different manufacturers' products (including generic products):

- *Category 3*: it is usually unnecessary to ensure that patients are maintained on a specific manufacturer's product unless there are specific concerns, such as patient anxiety and risk of confusion/dosing error.

Indications

Epilepsy
Adjunctive therapy of focal seizures with and without secondary generalization.

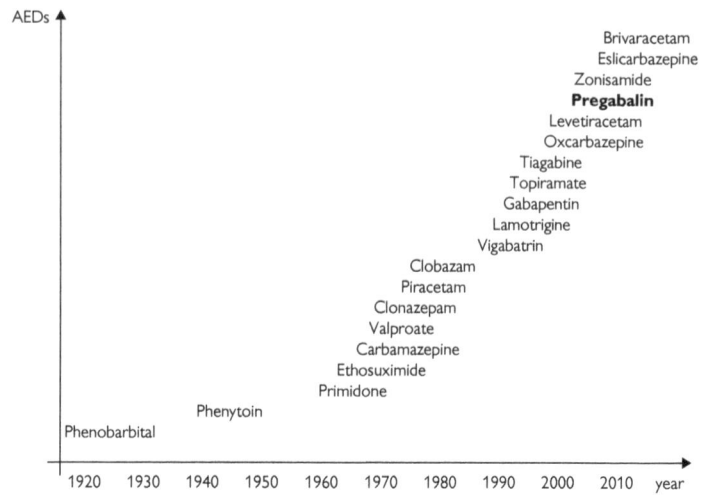

Fig. 11.1 Chronology of the clinical use of pregabalin

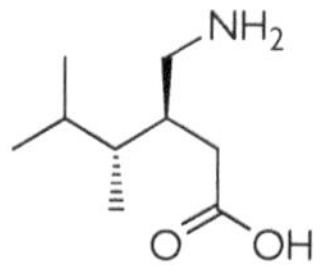

Fig. 11.2 Chemical structure of pregabalin

This figure is licensed under the Creative Commons Attribution-Share Alike 4.0 International license, https://creativecommons.org/licenses/by-sa/4.0/deed.en

Recommendations summarized from NICE (2012)

- *Seizure types*—on referral to tertiary care (focal seizures), contraindicated (generalized tonic-clonic seizures, tonic/atonic seizures, absence seizures, myoclonic seizures).
- *Epilepsy types*—on referral to tertiary care (benign epilepsy with centrotemporal spikes, panayiotopoulos syndrome, late-onset childhood occipital epilepsy), contraindicated (absence syndromes, idiopathic generalized epilepsy, juvenile myoclonic epilepsy, Dravet syndrome, Lennox–Gastaut syndrome).

Psychiatry

Generalized anxiety disorder.

Neurology

Peripheral and central neuropathic pain.

Dose titration

- *Epilepsy—adjunctive therapy*: 25 mg bd for 7 days, to be increased by 50 mg every 7days; usual maintenance 300 mg daily, divided into 2 or 3 doses (max. 600 mg daily, divided into 2 or 3 doses).
- *Generalized anxiety disorder*: 150 mg daily, divided into 2 or 3 doses, for 7 days, to be increased by 150 mg every 7 days (max. 600 mg daily, divided into 2 or 3 doses).

If stopping pregabalin, it is recommended to taper over at least 1 week to avoid abrupt withdrawal.

Plasma levels monitoring

Pregabalin pharmacokinetics are linear over the recommended daily dose range; inter-subject pharmacokinetic variability for pregabalin is low (<20%) and multiple dose pharmacokinetics are predictable from single-dose data. Therefore, there is no need for routine monitoring of plasma concentrations of pregabalin.

Cautions

- Patients with conditions that may precipitate encephalopathy.
- Patients with severe congestive heart failure.

Adverse effects

Pregabalin can be associated with adverse effects at the level of the nervous system and other systems (Table 11.1).

Interactions

- Since pregabalin is predominantly excreted unchanged in the urine, undergoes negligible metabolism in humans, does not inhibit drug metabolism in vitro, and is not bound to plasma proteins, it is unlikely to produce or be subject to pharmacokinetic interactions.
- Pregabalin may potentiate the effects of lorazepam.
- In the post-marketing experience, there are reports of respiratory failure and coma in patients taking pregabalin and other central nervous system depressant medicinal products. Pregabalin appears to be additive in the impairment of cognitive and gross motor function caused by oxycodone.

Table 11.1 Estimated frequency of adverse effects of pregabalin

Very common (>1 in 10 patients on pregabalin)	
Nervous system • dizziness • drowsiness • headache	*Other systems*

Common (>1 in 100 patients on pregabalin)	
Nervous system • amnesia • ataxia • blurred vision, visual field defects, and other visual disturbances • confusion • diplopia • euphoria • impaired attention • insomnia • irritability • paraesthesias • speech disorder	*Other systems* • appetite changes • constipation • dry mouth • flatulence • malaise • oedema • sexual dysfunction • vomiting • weight gain

Uncommon (>1 in 1000 patients on pregabalin)	
Nervous system • abnormal dreams • agitation • cognitive impairment • depersonalization • depression • hallucinations • hyperacusis • panic attacks • stupor • syncope • taste disturbance	*Other systems* • abdominal distension • arthralgia • chills • dry eye • dyspnoea • dysuria • first-degree atrio-ventricular block • flushing • gastro-oesophageal reflux disease • hypersalivation • hypertension • hypotension • lacrimation • myalgia • nasal dryness • nasopharyngitis • rash • sweating • tachycardia • thirst • thrombocytopenia • urinary incontinence

Table 11.1 Continued	
Rare (>1 in 10,000 patients on pregabalin)	
Nervous system • dysphagia • parosmia	Other systems • arrhythmia • ascites • bradycardia • breast pain, hypertrophy, and discharge • cold extremities • cough • epistaxis • hyperglycaemia • hypokalaemia • leucopenia and neutropenia • menstrual disturbances • oliguria • pancreatitis • renal failure • rhabdomylisis • rhinitis • urticaria • weight loss
Very rare (<1 in 10,000 patients on pregabalin)	
Nervous system	Other systems

With alcohol/food

- There are no specific foods that must be excluded from diet when taking pregabalin.
- Pregabalin may potentiate the effects of alcohol.

Special populations

Hepatic impairment

No dose adjustment is required for patients with hepatic impairment.

Renal impairment

Reduce maintenance dose according to degree of reduction in creatinine clearance.

Pregnancy

- There is no adequate data from the use of pregabalin in pregnant women. The potential risk for reproductive toxicity in humans is unknown. Pregabalin should not be used during pregnancy unless the benefit to the mother clearly outweighs the potential risk to the foetus.

- Pregabalin is excreted into human milk. The effect of pregabalin on newborns/infants is unknown. A case-by-case decision must be made whether to discontinue breast-feeding or to discontinue pregabalin therapy taking into account the benefit of breastfeeding for the child and the benefit of therapy for the woman.

Behavioural and cognitive effects in patients with epilepsy

Pregalin is characterized by a good behavioural profile. This AED does not appear to have significant negative effects on mood or behaviour in patients with epilepsy, although depression has been reported in some patients (dose-dependent effects of mild-to-moderate intensity). A potential abuse or misuse of pregabalin has also been reported, with implications in terms of dependence and withdrawal. Pregabalin is also associated with limited negative cognitive effects, mainly related to sedation, decreased arousal, decreased attention and concentration (dose-dependent effects of mild-to-moderate intensity).

Psychiatric use

Pregabalin has an approved indication and is widely used for the treatment of generalized anxiety disorder. Several randomized, double-blind, placebo-controlled trials found that pregabalin is an effective treatment for patients with

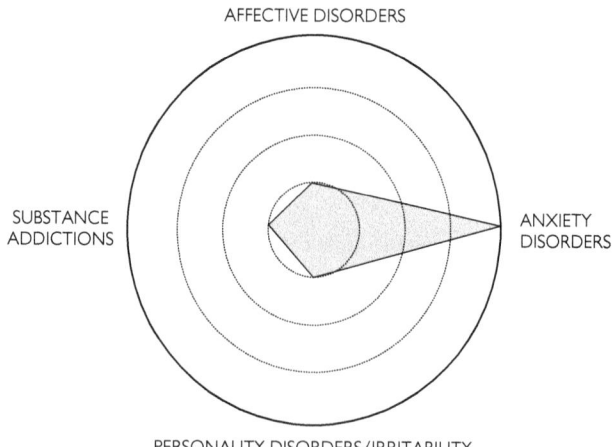

Fig. 11.3 Level of evidence supporting the psychiatric use of pregabalin in patients with behavioural symptoms

generalized anxiety disorder and social anxiety disorder. Possible implications in the treatment of mood disorders and benzodiazepines dependence are emerging. Moreover, pregabalin may be a therapeutic agent for the treatment of alcohol abuse, in both withdrawal phase and relapse prevention (Fig. 11.3).

Overall rating

Pregabalin is characterized by few antiepileptic indications, with a very good interaction profile in polytherapy; it has a very good behavioural tolerability profile and a wide range of psychiatric uses (Table 11.2).

Table 11.2 Overall rating of pregabalin	
Antiepileptic indications	☺
Interactions in polytherapy	☺ ☺ ☺
Behavioural tolerability	☺ ☺ ☺
Psychiatric use	☺ ☺ ☺
Key: ☺ ☺ ☺ = very good; ☺ ☺ = good; ☺ = acceptable.	

CHAPTER 12

Tiagabine

Tiagabine is a second-generation antiepileptic drug (AED; Fig. 12.1) known under the proprietary brand name of Gabitril® (Teva, Petah Tikva, Israel) in the UK and USA (Fig. 12.2).

Preparations

Tablets
- Tiagabine 5 mg (100-tab pack).
- Tiagabine 10 mg (100-tab pack).
- Tiagabine 15 mg (100-tab pack).

Generic formulation

MHRA/CHM advice to minimize risk when switching patients with epilepsy between different manufacturers' products (including generic products):

- *Category 3*: it is usually unnecessary to ensure that patients are maintained on a specific manufacturer's product unless there are specific concerns, such as patient anxiety and risk of confusion/dosing error.

Indications

Epilepsy: adjunctive therapy for focal seizures with or without secondary generalization that are not satisfactorily controlled by other AEDs.

Recommendations summarized from NICE (2012)

- *Seizure types*: on referral to tertiary care (focal seizures), contraindicated (generalized tonic-clonic seizures, tonic/atonic seizures, absence seizures, myoclonic seizures).
- *Epilepsy types*: on referral to tertiary care (benign epilepsy with centrotemporal spikes, panayiotopoulos syndrome, late-onset childhood occipital epilepsy), contraindicated (absence syndromes, idiopathic generalized epilepsy, juvenile myoclonic epilepsy, Dravet syndrome, Lennox–Gastaut syndrome).

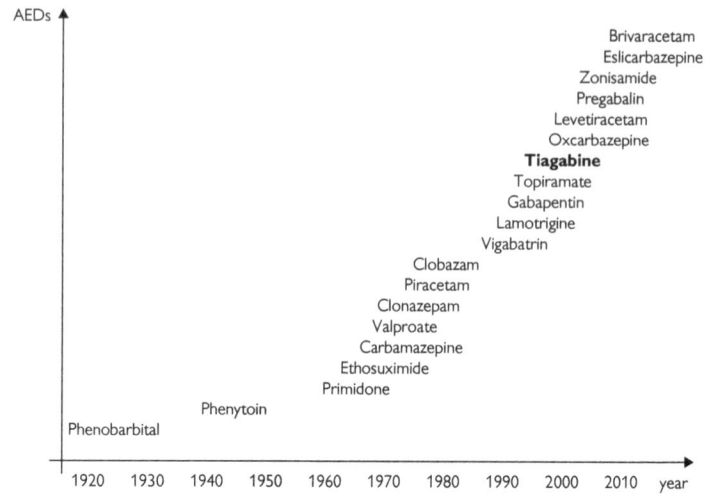

Fig. 12.1 Chronology of the clinical use of tiagabine

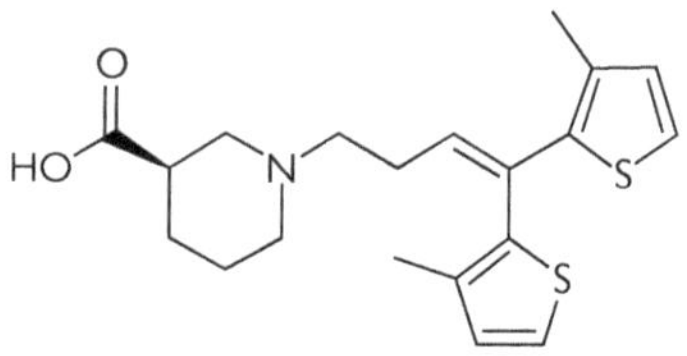

Fig. 12.2 Chemical structure of tiagabine

Dose titration

- *Epilepsy—adjunctive therapy (with enzyme-inducing AEDs):* 5–10 mg daily divided into 1 or 2 doses for 7 days, then increased by 5–10 mg daily every 7 days; usual maintenance 30–45 mg daily divided into 2 or 3 doses.
- *Epilepsy—adjunctive therapy (without enzyme-inducing AEDs):* 5–10 mg daily divided into 1 or 2 doses for 7 days, then increased by 5–10 mg daily every 7 days; usual maintenance 30–45 mg daily divided into 2–3 doses.

Plasma levels monitoring

The inter-individual variation in liver metabolism makes tiagabine a strong candidate for therapeutic drug monitoring. A broad reference range of 20–200 ng/mL has been proposed, however, the relatively short half-life of tiagabine under most conditions means that care must be taken in drawing blood for therapeutic drug monitoring. The high binding to serum proteins further suggests that measurement of free drug concentrations may be useful. However, there has been little investigation of the relationship between serum/plasma concentrations and therapeutic efficacy.

Cautions

- Patients with acute porphyrias.
- Patients with absence, myoclonic, tonic and atonic seizures (risk of exacerbation).

Adverse effects

Tiagabine can be associated with adverse effects at the level the nervous system and other systems (Table 12.1).

Table 12.1 Estimated frequency of adverse effects of tiagabine	
Very common (>1 in 10 patients on tiagabine)	
Nervous system • dizziness • nervousness • tiredness • tremor	Other systems • nausea
Common (>1 in 100 patients on tiagabine)	
Nervous system • anxiety • emotional lability • impaired concentration • speech impairment	Other systems • diarrhoea
Uncommon (>1 in 1000 patients on tiagabine)	
Nervous system	Other systems
Rare (>1 in 10,000 patients on tiagabine)	
Nervous system • confusion • depression • drowsiness • non-convulsive status epilepticus • psychosis • suicidal ideation • visual disturbances	Other systems
Very rare (<1 in 10,000 patients on tiagabine)	
Nervous system	Other systems

Interactions

With AEDs

- AEDs that induce hepatic enzymes (such as carbamazepine, phenytoin, phenobarbital, and primidone) enhance the metabolism of tiagabine: the plasma concentration of tiagabine may be reduced by a factor 1.5–3 by concomitant use of these AEDs.
- Tiagabine reduces the plasma concentration of valproate by about 10% (this is not considered clinically important and does not warrant a dose modification).

With other drugs

- Cimetidine increases the bioavailability of tiagabine by about 5% (this is not considered clinically important and does not warrant a dose modification).
- The combination of tiagabine with St John's wort (*Hypericum perforatum*) may lead to lower exposure and loss of efficacy of tiagabine, due to the potent induction of CYP3A4 by St John's wort, resulting in increased tiagabine metabolism. Therefore, the combination of tiagabine with St John's wort is contraindicated.

With alcohol/food

There are no known specific interactions between alcohol and tiagabine and there are no specific foods that must be excluded from diet when taking tiagabine. Administration with food results in a decreased rate and not extent of absorption

Special populations

Hepatic impairment

- Reduce dose, prolong the dose interval, or both, in mild to moderate impairment.
- Avoid in severe impairment.

Renal impairment

Renal insufficiency does not affect the pharmacokinetics of tiagabine, therefore its dosage does not need to be modified.

Pregnancy

- Clinical experience of the use of tiagabine in pregnant women is limited and no information on tiagabine during breastfeeding is available. Therefore, as a precautionary measure, it is preferable not to use tiagabine during

pregnancy or breast-feeding unless the potential benefits of treatment outweigh the potential risks.
- In case of tiagabine treatment during pregnancy, the dose should be monitored carefully and adjustments made on a clinical basis.

Behavioural and cognitive effects in patients with epilepsy

Treatment with tiagabine has often been associated with depression and irritability. Results from randomized double-blind, controlled trials with tiagabine as adjunctive treatment have confirmed the incidence of psychiatric problems, which can be mild-to-moderate in severity and can be reported more frequently by patients with a personal history of affective disorders, or in case of rapid initial titration. Tiagabine is characterized by a good profile in terms of cognitive adverse effects, with mild effects on concentration and memory, which can be minimized by slow initial titration.

Psychiatric use

Tiagabine has no approved indications in psychiatry and there is no conclusive evidence for its efficacy in the treatment of any behavioural problems (Fig. 12.3).

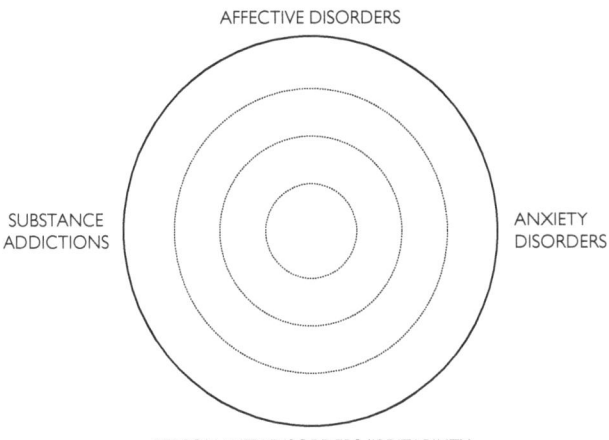

Fig. 12.3 Level of evidence supporting the psychiatric use of tiagabine in patients with behavioural symptoms

Overall rating

Tiagabine is characterized by few antiepileptic indications, with an acceptable interaction profile in polytherapy; it has an acceptable behavioural tolerability profile and no psychiatric uses (Table 12.2).

Table 12.2 Overall rating of tiagabine	
Antiepileptic indications	☺
Interactions in polytherapy	☺
Behavioural tolerability	☺
Psychiatric use	
Key: ☺☺☺ = very good; ☺☺ = good; ☺ = acceptable.	

CHAPTER 13

Topiramate

Topiramate is a second-generation antiepileptic drug (AED; Fig. 13.1) known by the proprietary brand name of Topamax® (Janssen-Cilag, High Wycombe) in the UK and USA (Raritan, NJ; Fig. 13.2).

Preparations

Tablets

- Topiramate 25 mg (60-tab pack).
- Topiramate 50 mg (60-tab pack).
- Topiramate 100 mg (60-tab pack).
- Topiramate 200 mg (60-tab pack).

Capsules

- Topiramate 15 mg (60-cap pack).
- Topiramate 25 mg (60-cap pack).
- Topiramate 50 mg (60-cap pack).

Generic formulation

MHRA/CHM advice to minimize risk when switching patients with epilepsy between different manufacturers' products (including generic products):

- *Category 2*: the need for continued supply of a particular manufacturer's product should be based on clinical judgment and consultation with the patient and/or carer taking into account factors such as seizure frequency and treatment history).

Indications

Epilepsy: monotherapy and adjunctive therapy of focal and generalized seizures.

Behavioural Neurology of Antiepileptic Drugs

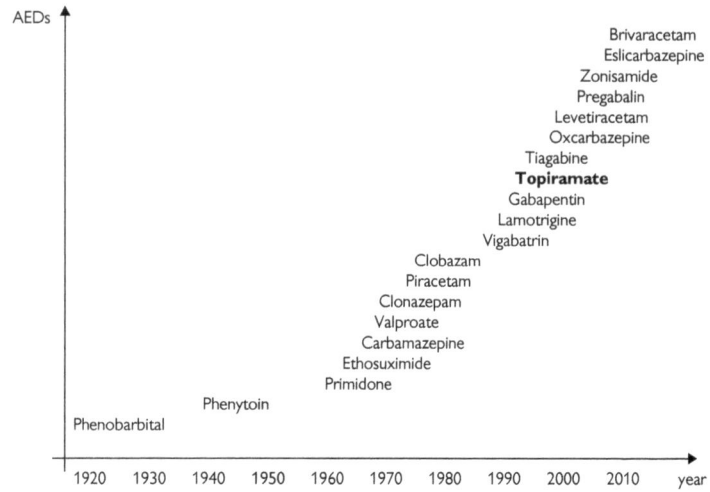

Fig. 13.1 Chronology of the clinical use of topiramate

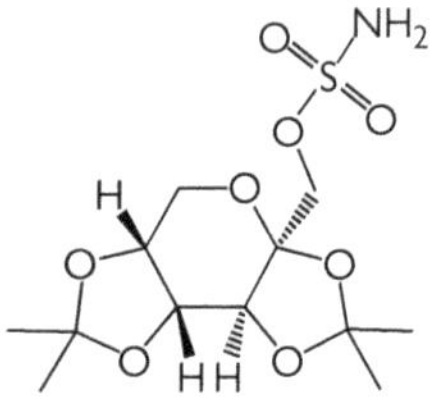

Fig. 13.2 Chemical structure of topiramate

Recommendations summarized from NICE (2012)

- *Seizure types*: first line (myoclonic seizures), adjunctive (generalized tonic-clonic seizures, focal seizures, myoclonic seizures), on referral to tertiary care (tonic/atonic seizures, absence seizures).
- *Epilepsy types*: first line (juvenile myoclonic epilepsy, idiopathic generalized epilepsy, Dravet), adjunctive (juvenile myoclonic epilepsy, epilepsy with generalized tonic-clonic seizures only, idiopathic generalized epilepsy, benign epilepsy with centrotemporal spikes, Panayiotopoulos syndrome, late-onset childhood occipital epilepsy), on referral to tertiary care (absence syndromes), contraindicated (Lennox–Gastaut syndrome).

Neurology: migraine prophylaxis

Dose titration

Epilepsy

Monotherapy

25 mg nocte for 7 days, then increased by 25–50 mg every 7–14 days; usual maintenance 100–200 mg daily divided into two doses (max 500 mg daily, although doses of 1000 mg daily have been used for refractory epilepsy).

Adjunctive therapy

25–50 mg nocte for 7 days then increased by 25–50 mg every 7–14 days; usual maintenance 200–400 mg daily divided into two doses (max 400 mg daily). In case of a missed dose, take the next dose; *do not* take an extra tablet to make up for the missed one.

Plasma levels monitoring

Topiramate is not a potent inducer of drug metabolizing enzymes, can be administered without regard to meals, and routine monitoring of plasma topiramate concentrations is not usually necessary. In clinical studies, there was no consistent relationship between plasma concentrations and efficacy or adverse events.

Cautions

- Patients with acute porphyrias.
- Patients with risk factors for metabolic acidosis.
- Patients with risk factors for nephrolithiasis (ensure adequate hydration).

Adverse effects

Topiramate can be associated with adverse effects at the level the nervous system and other systems (Table 13.1).

Table 13.1 Estimated frequency of adverse effects of topiramate

Very common (>1 in 10 patients on topiramate)	
Nervous system	*Other systems*
• depression	• diarrhoea
• dizziness	• nausea
• drowsiness	• weight loss
• fatigue	
• paraesthesias	

(*continued*)

Table 13.1 Continued	
Common (>1 in 100 patients on topiramate)	
Nervous system • aggression • agitation • anxiety • cognitive impairment • confusion • impaired attention • impaired coordination • irritability • mood changes • movement disorders • nystagmus • seizures • sleep disturbance • speech disorder • taste disturbance • tinnitus • tremor • visual disturbances	*Other systems* • abdominal pain • alopecia • anaemia • arthralgia • constipation • dry mouth • dyspepsia • dyspnoea • epistaxis • gastritis • malaise • muscle spasms, muscular weakness, and myalgia • nephrolithiasis • pruritus • skin rash • urinary disorders • vomiting
Uncommon (>1 in 1000 patients on topiramate)	
Nervous system • altered sense of smell • hearing loss • mydriasis • panic attacks • photophobia • psychosis • suicidal ideation • thirst	*Other systems* • abdominal distension • blepharospasm • blood disorders • bradycardia • dry eye • flatulence • flushing • gingival bleeding • glossodynia • haematuria • halitosis • hypokalaemia • hypotension and postural hypotension • increased lacrimation • influenza-like symptoms • leucopenia, neutropenia, thrombocytopenia • metabolic acidosis • palpitation • pancreatitis • peripheral neuropathy

Table 13.1 Continued	
	• reduced sweating • salivation • sexual dysfunction • skin discoloration • urinary calculus
Rare (>1 in 10,000 patients on topiramate)	
Nervous system • unilateral blindness	*Other systems* • abnormal skin odour • calcinosis • hepatic failure and hepatitis • periorbital oedema • Raynaud's syndrome • severe skin reaction (Stevens–Johnson syndrome)
Very rare (<1 in 10,000 patients on topiramate)	
Nervous system	*Other systems:* • angle-closure glaucoma*

*Acute myopia with secondary angle-closure glaucoma, typically occurring within 1 month of starting topiramate therapy. Choroidal effusions resulting in anterior displacement of the lens and iris have also been reported. I raised intra-ocular pressure occurs, it is recommended that the patient seek ophthalmological advice, use appropriate measures to reduce intra-ocular pressure, and stop topiramate as rapidly as possible.

Interactions

With AEDs

- Carbamazepine and phenytoin decrease the plasma concentration of topimarate. Therefore, the addition or withdrawal of carbamazepine and phenytoin to topiramate therapy may require an adjustment in dosage of the latter: this should be done by titrating to clinical effect.
- The addition of topiramate to phenytoin may result in an increase of plasma concentrations of phenytoin, possibly due to inhibition of a specific enzyme polymorphic isoform (CYP2C19). Therefore, any patient on phenytoin showing clinical signs or symptoms of toxicity should have phenytoin levels monitored.

With other drugs
Nil.

With alcohol/food

- Concomitant administration of topiramate and alcohol (or other CNS depressant drugs) has not been evaluated in clinical studies. it is recommended that topiramate not be used concomitantly with alcohol or other CNS depressant drugs.
- There are no specific foods that must be excluded from diet when taking topiramate.

Special populations

Hepatic impairment

Use with caution in moderate to severe impairment, as topiramate clearance may be reduced.

Renal impairment

In patients with impaired renal function topiramate should be administered with caution as the plasma and renal clearance of topiramate are decreased. Subjects with known renal impairment may require a longer time to reach steady-state at each dose. Half of the usual starting and maintenance dose is recommended.

Pregnancy

- Clinical data from pregnancy registries indicate that infants exposed to topiramate monotherapy have an increased risk (three-fold for topiramate monotherapy) of major congenital malformations (particularly cleft lip/palate, hypospadias, and anomalies involving various body systems) following exposure during the first trimester (increased risk of teratogenic effects associated with the use of AEDs in combination therapy).
- Clinical data from pregnancy registries indicate that infants exposed to topiramate monotherapy have a higher prevalence of low birth weight (<2500 g) compared with a reference group.
- It is therefore recommended that women of child-bearing age use highly effective contraception and consider alternative therapeutic options. In case of administration during the first trimester, careful prenatal monitoring should be performed. The dose of topiramate should be monitored carefully during pregnancy and after birth, and adjustments made on a clinical basis. It is recommended that the foetal growth is monitored.
- Although the excretion of topiramate in human milk has not been evaluated in controlled studies, limited observations in patients suggest an extensive excretion of topiramate into breast milk. Therefore, the options of suspending breastfeeding or discontinuing/abstaining from topiramate therapy should be carefully weighed up.

Behavioural and cognitive effects in patients with epilepsy

Treatment with topiramate has been associated with a number of negative behavioural effects in patients with epilepsy, in particular depression, irritability, and psychotic symptoms. Identified risk factors for the development of behavioural adverse effects include high starting doses and rapid titration schedules, as well as personal or family history of psychiatric disorders. The cognitive profile of topiramate is chacterized by fairly consistent evidence of adverse effects: in addition to attention, memory, and language (especially word-finding difficulties), confusion and psychomotor slowing have occasionally been reported. Most adverse cognitive effects occur at high doses and can be minimized by slow titration.

Psychiatric use

There is some evidence that topiramate may be effective in the treatment of depression, either as monotherapy or as adjunctive treatment. The findings of initial reports suggesting that topiramate can be effective in the treatment of bipolar disorder and post-traumatic stress disorders have not been confirmed by the results of randomized controlled trials. Preliminary data suggest some efficacy in Tourette syndrome, obsessive-compulsive disorder, eating disorders (binge eating), behavioural and psychological symptoms of dementia, alcohol and cocaine dependence. In late 2012, topiramate was approved by the USA FDA in

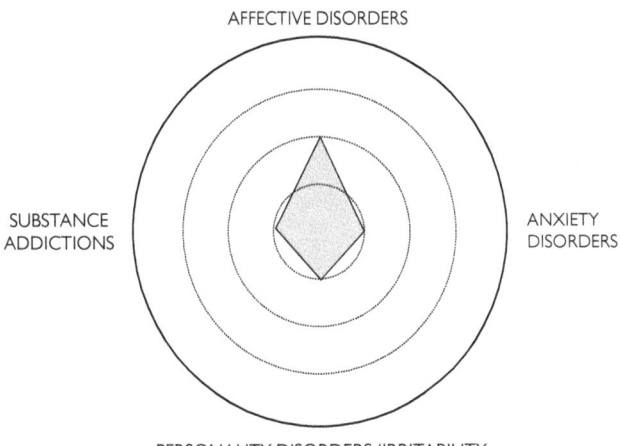

Fig. 13.3 Level of evidence supporting the psychiatric use of topiramate in patients with behavioural symptoms

combination with phentermine for weight loss: this is a clinically significant effect in patients with behavioural problems, as psychopharmacological treatment is often associated with metabolic dysfunction and weight gain (Fig. 13.3).

Overall rating

Topiramate is characterized by a good range of antiepileptic indications, with an acceptable interaction profile in polytherapy; it has an acceptable behavioural tolerability profile and a restricted range of psychiatric uses (Table 13.2).

Table 13.2 Overall rating of topiramate	
Antiepileptic indications	☺☺
Interactions in polytherapy	☺
Behavioural tolerability	☺
Psychiatric use	☺
Key: ☺☺☺ = very good; ☺☺ = good; ☺ = acceptable.	

CHAPTER 14

Valproate

Valproate is a first-generation antiepileptic drug (AED; Fig. 14.1) known with the proprietary brand names of Epilim® (Sanofi, Paris) and Episenta® (Desitin, Hamburg) in the UK and Depakote® (Sanofi, Paris) in the USA (Fig. 14.2).

Preparations

Tablets
Valproate 100 mg (100-tab pack).

Modified-release tablets
- Valproate 200 mg (100-tab pack).
- Valproate 300 mg (100-tab pack).
- Valproate 500 mg (100-tab pack).

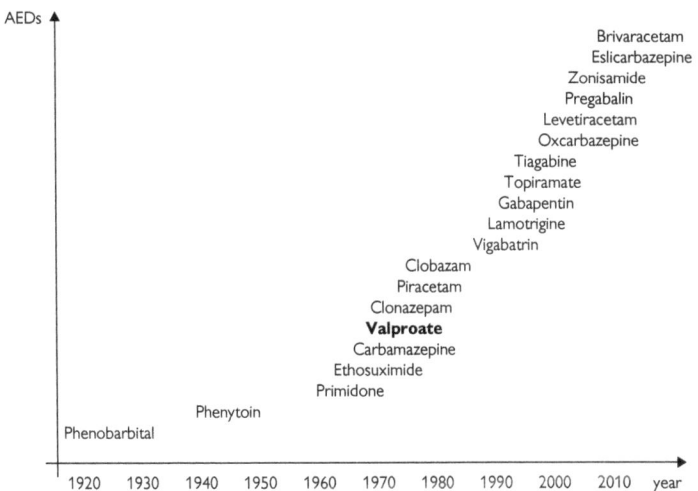

Fig. 14.1 Chronology of the clinical use of valproate

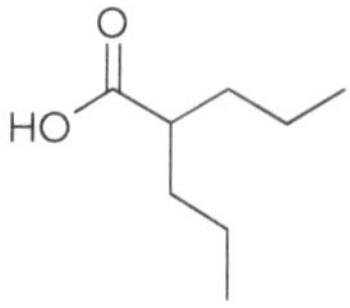

Fig. 14.2 Chemical structure of valproate

Gastro-resistant tablets
- Valproate 200 mg (100-tab pack).
- Valproate 500 mg (100-tab pack).

Modified-release capsules
- Valproate 150 mg (100-cap pack).
- Valproate 300 mg (100-cap pack).

Modified-release granules
- Valproate 50 mg (30-sachet pack).
- Valproate 100 mg (30-sachet pack).
- Valproate 250 mg (30-sachet pack).
- Valproate 500 mg (30-sachet pack).
- Valproate 750 mg (30-sachet pack).
- Valproate 1000 mg (30-sachet pack).

Oral solution
Valproate 40 mg/mL (300 mL).

Generic formulation

MHRA/CHM advice to minimize risk when switching patients with epilepsy between different manufacturers' products (including generic products):

- *Category 2*: the need for continued supply of a particular manufacturer's product should be based on clinical judgment and consultation with the patient and/or carer, taking into account factors such as seizure frequency and treatment history.

Indications

Epilepsy
Monotherapy and adjunctive therapy of focal and generalized seizures.

Recommendations summarized from NICE (2012)

- *Seizure types:* first line (generalized tonic-clonic seizures, tonic/atonic seizures, absence seizures, myoclonic seizures, focal seizures), adjunctive (generalized tonic-clonic seizures, absence seizures, myoclonic seizures, focal seizures).
- *Epilepsy types:* first line (absence syndromes, juvenile myoclonic epilepsy, epilepsy with generalized tonic-clonic seizures only, idiopathic generalized epilepsy, benign epilepsy with centrotemporal spikes, Panayiotopoulos syndrome, late-onset childhood occipital epilepsy, Dravet syndrome, Lennox–Gastaut syndrome), adjunctive (absence syndromes, juvenile myoclonic epilepsy, epilepsy with generalized tonic-clonic seizures only, idiopathic generalized epilepsy, benign epilepsy with centrotemporal spikes, panayiotopoulos syndrome, late-onset childhood occipital epilepsy).

Psychiatry
Treatment of acute mania associated with bipolar disorder.

Neurology
Migraine prophylaxis (unlicensed).

Dose titration

Epilepsy
600 mg daily divided into 1 or 2 doses, then increased by 150–300 mg every 3 days; usual maintenance 1000–2000 mg (or 20–30 mg/kg) daily divided into 1 or 2 doses (max 2500 mg daily).

Mania
750 mg daily divided into 1 or 2 doses, adjusted according to response; usual maintenance 1000–2000 mg daily divided into 1 or 2 doses (doses greater than 45 mg/kg daily require careful monitoring).

Plasma levels monitoring

Although plasma levels can be measured, and a therapeutic range has been postulated (40–100 mg/L), plasma valproate concentrations are not a useful index of efficacy. Therefore, routine monitoring is unhelpful.

Cautions

- Patients with systemic lupus erythematosus.
- Patients with a personal or family history of severe hepatic dysfunction (contraindication).
- Patients with known metabolic disorders (contraindication).

- Patients with suspected metabolic disorders (contraindication).
- Patients with porphyria (contraindication).

Adverse effects

Valproate can be associated with adverse effects at the level the nervous system and other systems (Table 14.1).

Table 14.1 Estimated frequency of adverse effects of valproate

Very common (>1 in 10 patients on valproate)	
Nervous system	*Other systems*
• tremor	• nausea
Common (>1 in 100 patients on valproate)	
Nervous system	*Other systems*
• aggression	• anaemia
• amnesia	• diarrhoea
• confusion	• gastric irritation
• convulsions	• haemorrhage
• deafness	• hyponatraemia
• drowsiness	• menstrual disturbance
• extrapyramidal disorders	• thrombocytopenia
• headache	• transient hair loss
• nystagmus	• weight gain
• stupor	
Uncommon (>1 in 1000 patients on valproate)	
Nervous system	*Other systems*
• ataxia	• angioedema
• coma	• leucopenia and pancytopenia
• encephalopathy	• peripheral oedema
• increased alertness	• skin rash
• lethargy	• reduced bone density
• paraesthesias	• syndrome of inappropriate secretion of antidiuretic hormone (SIADH)
	• vasculitis
Rare (>1 in 10,000 patients on valproate)	
Nervous system	*Other systems*
• disorders and dementia	• AED hypersensitivity syndrome (DRESS)
	• blood disorders
	• bone marrow failure
	• enuresis
	• Fanconi's syndrome
	• hyperammonaemia

Table 14.1 Continued	
	• hypothyroidism • male infertility • myelodysplastic syndrome • polycystic ovaries • severe skin reactions (Stevens–Johnson syndrome, toxic epidermal necrolysis)* • systemic lupus erythematosus
Very rare (<1 in 10,000 patients on valproate)	
Nervous system	Other systems • acne • gynaecomastia • hepatic dysfunction* • hirsutism • increase in bleeding time • pancreatitis

*Liver dysfunction, including fatal hepatic failure, has occurred in association with valproate, usually in the first 6 months of therapy, usually involving multiple AEDs (monitor liver function before therapy and during first 6 months, especially in patients most at risk; withdraw treatment immediately if persistent vomiting and abdominal pain, anorexia, jaundice, oedema, malaise, drowsiness, or loss of seizure control).

Interactions

With AEDs

- AEDs with enzyme inducing effect (including carbamazepine, phenobarbital, phenytoin) decrease valproate plasma concentrations.
- Valproate reduces the metabolism of lamotrigine and increases the lamotrigine mean half-life by nearly two fold. This interaction may lead to increased lamotrigine toxicity, in particular serious skin rashes.
- Valproate increases phenobarbital and primidone plasma concentrations with exacerbation of its adverse effects (sedation may occur).
- Valproate may potentiate toxic effects of carbamazepine.
- Valproate decreases phenytoin total plasma concentration, but displaces phenytoin from its plasma protein binding sites and reduces its hepatic catabolism, thereby increasing phenytoin free form with possible overdose symptoms.
- Concomitant administration of valproate and topiramate has been associated with encephalopathy and/or hyperammonaemia. In patients taking these two AEDs, careful monitoring of signs and symptoms is advised (especially in patients with pre-existing encephalopathy).

With other drugs

- Mefloquine and chloroquine increase valproate metabolism and may lower the seizure threshold (therefore, epileptic seizures may occur in cases of combined therapy).
- Decreases in blood levels of valproate have been reported when it is co-administered with carbapenem antibiotics (such as imipenem, panipenem, meropenem), resulting in a 60–100% decrease in valproate levels within 2 days, sometimes associated with convulsions.
- Colestyramine may decrease the absorption of valproate.
- Rifampicin may decrease valproate blood levels, resulting in a lack of therapeutic effect.
- In case of concomitant use of valproate and highly protein bound agents (e.g. aspirin), free valproate plasma levels may be increased.
- Valproic acid plasma levels may be increased (as a result of reduced hepatic metabolism) in case of concomitant use with cimetidine or erythromycin.
- Valproate may potentiate the effect of other psychotropics such as antipsychotics (especially olanzapine), MAO inhibitors, antidepressants, and benzodiazepines.
- Valproate may raise zidovudine plasma concentration, possibly leading to increased zidovudine toxicity.
- The anticoagulant effect of warfarin and other coumarin anticoagulants may be increased following displacement from plasma protein binding sites by valproate.

With alcohol/food

There are no specific foods that must be excluded from diet when taking valproate. Alcohol intake is not recommended during treatment with valproate.

Special populations

Hepatic impairment

Avoid if possible: hepatotoxicity and hepatic failure may occasionally occur (usually in first 6 months). Avoid in active liver disease.

Renal impairment

In patients with renal insufficiency, it may be necessary to decrease dosage of valproate. As monitoring of plasma concentrations may be misleading, dosage should be adjusted according to clinical monitoring.

Pregnancy
- Valproate is associated with the highest risk of major and minor congenital malformations (in particular neural tube defects) and neurodevelopmental effects among AEDs.
- Therefore, valproate should not be used during pregnancy or in women of child-bearing age unless there is no safer alternative and only after a careful discussion of the risks.
- If valproate is to be used during pregnancy, the lowest effective dose should be prescribed in divided doses or as modified-release tablets to avoid peaks in plasma valproate concentrations (doses greater than 1000 mg daily are associated with an increased risk of teratogenicity). The dose should be monitored carefully during pregnancy and after birth, and adjustments made on a clinical basis.
- Avoid use in the treatment of epilepsy and bipolar disorder unless there is no safer alternative and only after a careful discussion of the risks (effective contraception advised in women of child-bearing potential).
- Neonatal bleeding (related to hypofibrinaemia) and hepatotoxicity have been reported, and specialist prenatal monitoring should be instigated when valproate has been taken in pregnancy.
- Valproate is excreted in human milk with a concentration ranging from 1 to 10% of maternal serum levels. Haematological disorders have been shown in breastfed newborns/infants of treated women. A decision must be made whether to discontinue breastfeeding or to discontinue/abstain from valproate therapy, taking into account the benefit of breastfeeding for the child and the benefit of therapy for the woman.

Behavioural and cognitive effects in patients with epilepsy

The incidence of adverse psychiatric effects associated with valproate in patients with epilepsy is overall negligible (apart from reports of depression, irritability, and other behavioural symptoms in the context of encephalopathy). Cognitive difficulties have occasionally been reported in patients with epilepsy treated with valproate, especially affecting attention and memory functions.

Psychiatric use

Valproate is an effective mood stabilizer, licensed for the treatment of acute mania in patients with bipolar disorder. Although it has no formal indication, it is also considered a first-line agent for maintenance treatment in bipolar disorder. There is evidence suggesting efficacy of valproate in the treatment of hostility

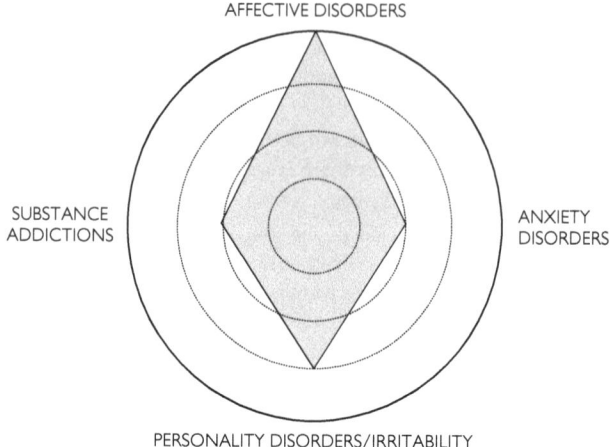

Fig. 14.3 Level of evidence supporting the psychiatric use of valproate in patients with behavioural symptoms

among patients with acute alcohol-associated hallucinosis or schizophrenia, and in impulsive/aggressive behaviours, either in isolation or in the context of co-morbid bipolar disorder or personality disorder. Available data show a limited efficacy of valproate in depressive disorders, schizophrenia, pathological gambling, as well as benzodiazepine/cannabis/cocaine dependence and acute alcohol withdrawal (Fig. 14.3).

Overall rating

Valproate is characterized by a wide range of antiepileptic indications, with an acceptable interaction profile in polytherapy; it has a good behavioural tolerability profile and a wide range of psychiatric uses (Table 14.2).

Table 14.2 Overall rating of valproate	
Antiepileptic indications	☺ ☺ ☺
Interactions in polytherapy	☺
Behavioural tolerability	☺ ☺
Psychiatric use	☺ ☺ ☺
Key: ☺ ☺ ☺ = very good; ☺ ☺ = good; ☺ = acceptable.	

CHAPTER 15

Vigabatrin

Vigabatrin is a second-generation anti-epileptic drug (AED; Fig. 15.1), known under the proprietary brand name of Sabril® (Sanofi, Paris) in the UK and USA (Fig. 15.2).

Preparations

Tablets

Vigabatrin 500 mg (100-tab pack).

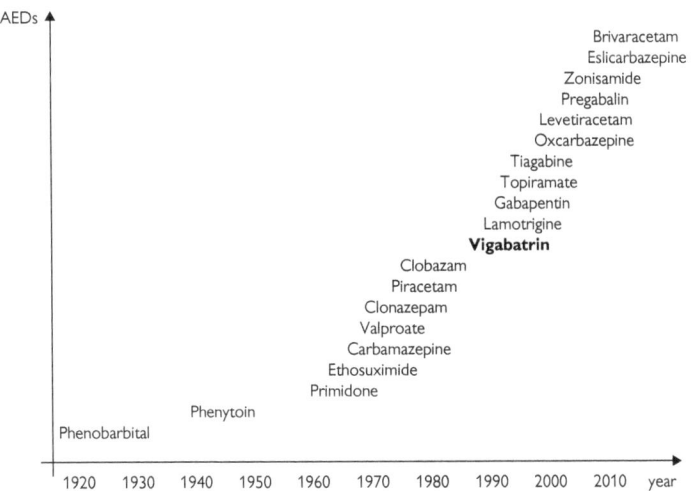

Fig. 15.1 Chronology of the clinical use of vigabatrin

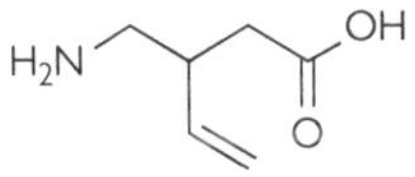

Fig. 15.2 Chemical structure of vigabatrin

Powder

Vigabatrin 500 mg (50-sachet pack).

Generic formulation

MHRA/CHM advice to minimize risk when switching patients with epilepsy between different manufacturers' products (including generic products):

- *Category 3*: it is usually unnecessary to ensure that patients are maintained on a specific manufacturer's product unless there are specific concerns, such as patient anxiety and risk of confusion/dosing error.

Indications

Epilepsy: adjunctive therapy of focal seizures with or without secondary generalization not satisfactorily controlled with other AEDs.

Recommendations summarized from NICE (2012)

- *Seizure types*: on referral to tertiary care (focal seizures), contraindicated (generalized tonic-clonic seizures, tonic/atonic seizures, absence seizures, myoclonic seizures).
- *Epilepsy types*: on referral to tertiary care (benign epilepsy with centrotemporal spikes, panayiotopoulos syndrome, late-onset childhood occipital epilepsy), contraindicated (absence syndromes, idiopathic generalized epilepsy, juvenile myoclonic epilepsy, Dravet syndrome, Lennox–Gastaut syndrome).

Dose titration

Epilepsy

Adjunctive therapy: 1000 mg daily divided into 1 or 2 doses for 7 days, then increased by 500 mg 7 days; usual maintenance 2000–3000 mg daily (max. 3000 mg daily).

Plasma levels monitoring

No direct correlation exists between the plasma concentration and the efficacy of vigabatrin. The duration of the effect of the medicinal product is dependent on the rate of GABA transaminase re-synthesis, rather than the concentration of the drug in the plasma. The routine measurement of plasma levels in clinical practice is therefore, unnecessary.

Cautions

- Patients with a history of behavioural problems, depression, psychosis.
- Elderly patients.
- Patients with visual field defects (contraindication).

Adverse effects

Vigabatrin can be associated with adverse effects at the level the nervous system and other systems (Table 15.1).

Table 15.1 Estimated frequency of adverse effects of vigabatrin	
Very common (>1 in 10 patients on vigabatrin)	
Nervous system • drowsiness • fatigue	*Other systems* • arthralgia
Common (>1 in 100 patients on vigabatrin)	
Nervous system • aggression • agitation • amnesia • blurred vision • depression • diplopia • dizziness • headache • impaired concentration • irritability • nystagmus • paraesthesias • paranoia • speech disorder • tremor • visual field defects*	*Other systems* • abdominal pain • nausea and vomiting • oedema • weight gain
Uncommon (>1 in 1000 patients on vigabatrin)	
Nervous system: - Ataxia - Mania - Increase in seizure frequency (especially myoclonic seizures) - Psychosis	Other systems: - Rash

(continued)

Table 15.1 Continued	
Rare (>1 in 10,000 patients on vigabatrin)	
Nervous system	Other systems
• encephalopathic symptoms (sedation, stupor, and confusion with non-specific slow wave EEG) • peripheral retinal neuropathy and other retinal disorders • suicidal ideation	
Very rare (<1 in 10,000 patients on vigabatrin)	
Nervous system • hepatitis • optic atrophy and optic neuritis	Other systems
*About one-third of patients treated with vigabatrin have suffered visual field defects: counselling and careful monitoring for this adverse effect is required. The onset of symptoms varies from 1 month to several years after starting vigabatrin; in most cases, visual field defects persist despite discontinuation, and further deterioration after discontinuation cannot be excluded. Visual field testing before treatment and at 6-month interval is recommended and gradual withdrawal of vigabatrin should be considered if visual field deficits are detected.	

Interactions

With AEDs

As vigabatrin is neither metabolized, nor protein bound and is not an inducer of hepatic cytochrome P450 drug metabolizing-enzymes, there are no significant interactions with other drugs. Controlled clinical studies have shown a gradual reduction of 16–33% in the plasma concentration of phenytoin (unlikely to be of therapeutic significance).

With other drugs

Nil.

With alcohol/food

There are no known specific interactions between alcohol and vigabatrin and there are no specific foods that must be excluded from diet when taking vigabatrin (food administration does not alter the extent of vigabatrin absorption).

Special populations

Hepatic impairment

No dose adjustment is required for patients with hepatic impairment.

Renal impairment
Consider reducing maintenance dose or frequency of administration.

Pregnancy
- Based on data on pregnancies exposed to vigabatrin, no definite conclusion can be drawn as to whether vigabatrin produces an increased risk of malformation when taken during pregnancy because of limited data and the administration of concomitant AEDs.
- Vigabatrin should not be used during pregnancy unless it is required based on the clinical condition of the patient. In such cases, the dose of vigabatrin should be monitored carefully during pregnancy and after birth, and adjustments made on a clinical basis.
- Vigabatrin is excreted in human milk: since there is insufficient information on the effects of vigabatrin in newborns/infants, the possibility of avoiding breast-feeding should be considered.

Behavioural and cognitive effects in patients with epilepsy

Patients treated with vigabatrin often report behavioural adverse effects (most frequently depression, psychosis, and irritability). Risk factors for developing adverse psychiatric effects during vigabatrin therapy include high starting and maintenance doses, past psychiatric history and epilepsy severity. Vigabatrin is characterized by

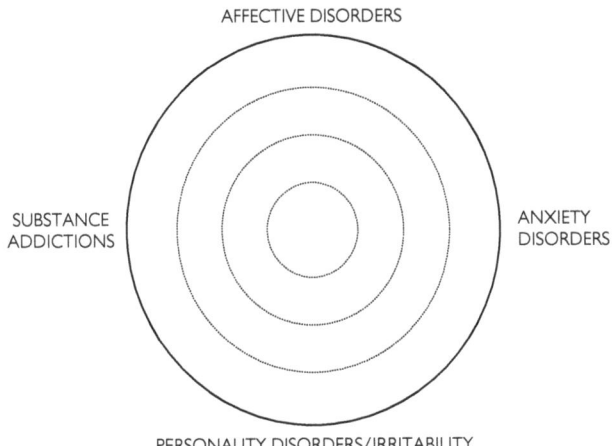

Fig. 15.3 Level of evidence supporting the psychiatric use of vigabatrin in patients with behavioural symptoms

a positive cognitive profile, with rare reports of memory, attention, and language problems.

Psychiatric use

Vigabatrin has no approved indications in psychiatry. There is weak evidence for usefulness in the treatment of anxiety disorders and addictions (Fig. 15.3).

Overall rating

Vigabatrin is characterized by a few antiepileptic indications, with a very good interaction profile in polytherapy; it has an acceptable behavioural tolerability profile and no psychiatric uses (Table 15.2).

Table 15.2 Overall rating of vigabatrin	
Antiepileptic indications	☺
Interactions in polytherapy	☺ ☺ ☺
Behavioural tolerability	☺
Psychiatric use	
Key: ☺ ☺ ☺ = very good; ☺ ☺ = good; ☺ = acceptable.	

CHAPTER 16

Zonisamide

Zonisamide is a second-generation antiepileptic drug (AED) (Fig. 16.1) known with the proprietary brand name of Zonegran® (Eisai) in the UK and USA (Fig. 16.2).

Preparations

Capsules

- Zonisamide 25 mg (14-tab pack).
- Zonisamide 50 mg (56-tab pack).
- Zonisamide 100 mg (56-tab pack).

Generic formulation

MHRA/CHM advice to minimize risk when switching patients with epilepsy between different manufacturers' products (including generic products):

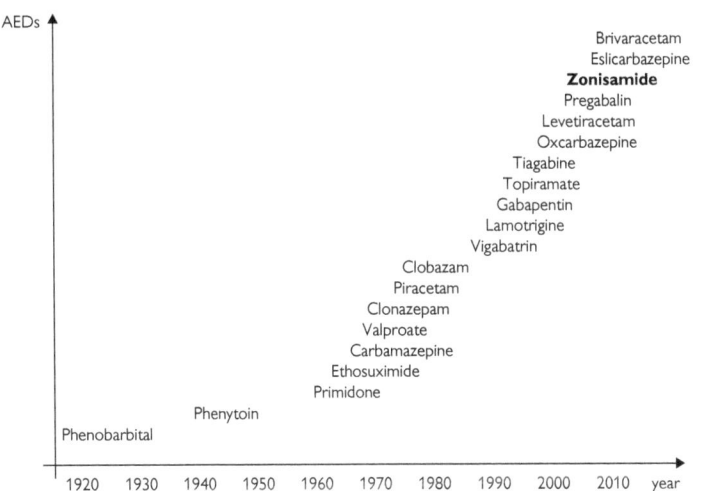

Fig. 16.1 Chronology of the clinical use of zonisamide

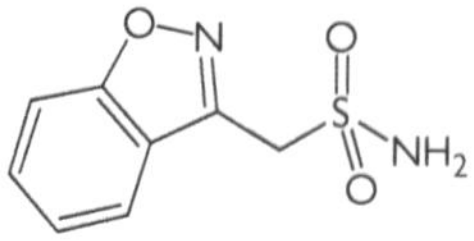

Fig. 16.2 Chemical structure of zonisamide

- *Category 2*: the need for continued supply of a particular manufacturer's product should be based on clinical judgment and consultation with the patient and/or carer taking into account factors such as seizure frequency and treatment history.

Indications

Epilepsy

Monotherapy of focal seizures with or without secondary generalization and adjunctive therapy of refractory focal seizures with or without secondary generalization.

Recommendations summarized from NICE (2012)

- *Seizure types*: on referral to tertiary care (absence seizures, focal seizures, myoclonic seizures).
- *Epilepsy types*: on referral to tertiary care (absence syndromes, juvenile myoclonic epilepsy, idiopathic generalized epilepsy, benign epilepsy with centrotemporal spikes, panayiotopoulos syndrome, late-onset childhood occipital epilepsy).

Dose titration

Epilepsy

Monotherapy

100 mg od for 14 days, then increased by 100 mg every 14 days; usual maintenance 300 mg od (max. 500 mg daily).

Adjunctive therapy

25 mg bd for 7 days, 50 mg bd for 7 days, then increased by 100 mg every 7 days; usual maintenance 300–500 mg daily, divided into 1 or 2 doses (dose to be increased every 14 days in patients who are not on carbamazepine, phenobarbital, phenytoin, or other potent inducers of cytochrome P450 enzyme CYP3A4).

Plasma levels monitoring

Although plasma levels can be measured, and a therapeutic range has been postulated (10–40 mg/L), there is little evidence base for recommending routine measurement of plasma levels in clinical practice.

Cautions

- Patients with metabolic acidosis (consider dose reduction or discontinuation if metabolic acidosis develops).
- Patients with low body weight or poor appetite (monitor weight throughout treatment).
- Patients with risk factors or predisposition to nephrolithiasis.
- Elderly patients.

Adverse effects

Zonisamide can be associated with adverse effects at the level the nervous system and other systems (Table 16.1).

Table 16.1 Estimated frequency of adverse effects of zonisamide

Very common (>1 in 10 patients on zonisamide)	
Nervous system • agitation • anorexia • ataxia • confusion • depression • diplopia • dizziness • drowsiness • irritability • memory problems	*Other systems*
Common (>1 in 100 patients on zonisamide)	
Nervous system • fatigue • impaired attention • insomnia • nystagmus • paraesthesias • psychosis • speech disorder • tremor	*Other systems* • abdominal pain • constipation • diarrhoea • ecchymosis • nausea • peripheral oedema • pruritus • pyrexia • skin rash (consider withdrawal)

(*continued*)

Table 16.1 Continued

Uncommon (>1 in 1000 patients on zonisamide)	
Nervous system • aggression • suicidal ideation • worsening of seizures	Other systems • cholecystitis and cholelithiasis • dyspepsia • hypokalaemia • pneumonia • urinary calculus and urinary tract infection • vomiting
Rare (>1 in 10,000 patients on zonisamide)	
Nervous system	Other systems
Very rare (<1 in 10,000 patients on zonisamide)	
Nervous system • amnesia • coma • hallucinations • myasthenic syndrome • neuroleptic malignant syndrome	Other systems • aspiration • blood disorders • dyspnoea • heat stroke • hepatitis • hydronephrosis • impaired sweating • metabolic acidosis • pancreatitis • renal failure and renal tubular acidosis • rhabdomyolysis • severe skin reactions (toxic epidermal necrolysis and Stevens–Johnson syndrome)

Interactions

With AEDs

- Exposure to zonisamide is lower in epileptic patients receiving CYP3A4-inducing agents such as phenytoin, carbamazepine, and phenobarbital. These effects are unlikely to be of clinical significance when zonisamide is added to existing therapy; however, changes in zonisamide concentrations may occur if concomitant CYP3A4-inducing antiepileptic or other medicinal products are withdrawn, dose adjusted or introduced, an adjustment of the zonisamide dose may be required.
- Zonisamide should be used with caution in adult patients treated concomitantly with carbonic anhydrase inhibitors such as topiramate and acetazolamide, as there are insufficient data to rule out a possible pharmacodynamic interaction.

With other drugs

- Caution is advised when starting or stopping zonisamide treatment or changing the zonisamide dose in patients who are also receiving P-gp substrates such as digoxin and quinidine.
- If co-administration with rifampicin (a potent CYP3A4 inducer) is necessary, the patient should be closely monitored and the dose of zonisamide and other CYP3A4 substrates adjusted as needed.

With alcohol/food

There are no known specific interactions between alcohol and zonisamide and there are no specific foods that must be excluded from diet when taking zonisamide.

Special populations

Hepatic impairment

- Initially increase dose every 14 days in moderate impairment.
- Avoid in severe impairment.

Renal impairment

- Initially increase dose every 14 days in moderate impairment.
- Discontinue if renal function deteriorates.

Pregnancy

- There are limited data from the use of zonisamide in pregnant women and the potential risk in terms of reproductive toxicity for humans is unknown.
- Zonisamide must not be used during pregnancy unless it is required based on the clinical condition of the patient. In such cases, the dose of zonisamide should be monitored carefully during pregnancy and after birth, and adjustments made on a clinical basis.
- Zonisamide is excreted in human milk; the concentration in breastmilk is similar to maternal plasma. A decision must be made whether to discontinue breastfeeding or to discontinue/abstain from zonisamide therapy. Due to the long retention time of zonisamide in the body, breastfeeding must not be resumed until 1 month after zonisamide therapy is completed.

Behavioural and cognitive effects in patients with epilepsy

The behavioural profile of zonisamide in patients with epilepsy features specific problems, which can occur with high doses. The most commonly reported behavioural symptoms are depression, irritability, agitation, and psychosis. Cognitive deficits reported by patients treated with zonisamide mainly involve attention, concentration, and language domains (most effects occur at high doses).

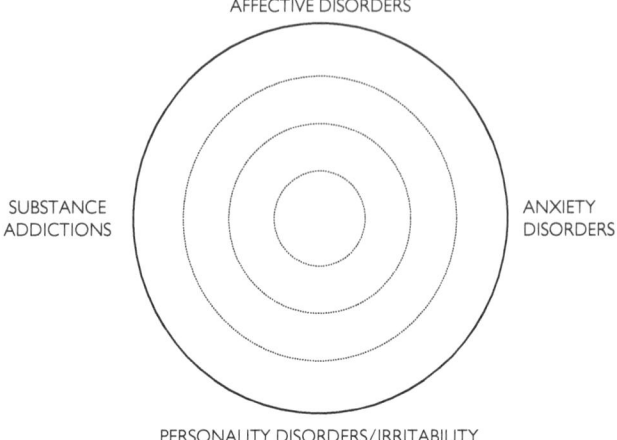

Fig. 16.3 Level of evidence supporting the psychiatric use of zonisamide in patients with behavioural symptoms

Psychiatric use

Zonisamide does not have any approved indications in psychiatry. Initial findings from uncontrolled studies suggesting that zonisamide may be effective in the treatment of bipolar disorder did not find confirmation. There is preliminary evidence for possible usefulness of zonisamide in the treatment of obesity and psychotropic-associated weight gain, as well as alcohol dependence and withdrawal (Fig. 16.3).

Overall rating

Zonisamide is characterized by a few antiepileptic indications, with an acceptable interaction profile in polytherapy; it has an acceptable tolerability profile and no psychiatric uses (Table 16.2).

Table 16.2 Overall rating of zonisamide	
Antiepileptic indications	☺
Interactions in polytherapy	☺
Behavioural tolerability	☺
Psychiatric use	
Key: ☺☺☺ = very good; ☺☺ = good; ☺ = acceptable.	

CHAPTER 17

Other antiepileptic drugs: rufinamide, lacosamide, perampanel

Rufinamide (licensed in 2007) is a third-generation AED known with the proprietary brand name of Invelon® (Eisai, Hatfield) in the UK and USA (Fig. 17.1). Lacosamide (licensed in 2008) is a third-generation AED known with the proprietary brand name of Vimpat® (UCB Pharma, Slough) in the UK and USA (Fig. 17.2). Perampanel (licensed in 2012) is a third-generation AED known with the proprietary brand name of Fycompa® (Eisai, Hatfield) in the UK and Banzel® (Eisai, Hatfield) in the USA (Fig. 17.3).

Preparations

Rufinamide

Tablets

- Rufinamide 100 mg (10-tab pack).
- Rufinamide 200 mg (60-tab pack).
- Rufinamide 400 mg (60-tab pack).

Oral suspension

Rufinamide 40 mg/mL (460 mL).

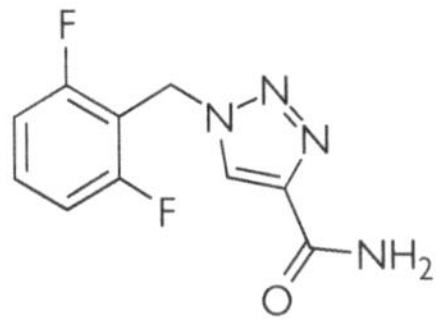

Fig. 17.1 Chronology of the clinical use of rufinamide

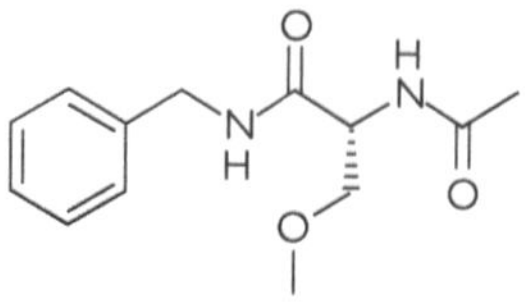

Fig. 17.2 Chronology of the clinical use of lacosamide

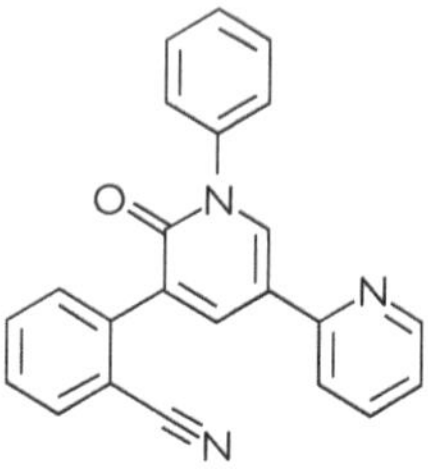

Fig. 17.3 Chronology of the clinical use of perampanel

Lacosamide

Tablets

- Lacosamide 50 mg (14-tab pack).
- Lacosamide 100 mg (14-tab pack).
- Lacosamide 150 mg (14-tab pack).
- Lacosamide 200 mg (56-tab pack).

Oral solution

Lacosamide 10mg/mL (200mL)

Perampanel

Tablets

- Perampanel 2 mg (7-tab pack).
- Perampanel 4 mg (28-tab pack).
- Perampanel 6 mg (28-tab pack).
- Perampanel 8 mg (28-tab pack).
- Perampanel 10 mg (28-tab pack).
- Perampanel 12 mg (28-tab pack).

OTHER ANTIEPILEPTIC DRUGS • 137

Generic formulation

Rufinamide, perampanel

MHRA/CHM advice to minimize risk when switching patients with epilepsy between different manufacturers' products (including generic products):

- *Category 2*: the need for continued supply of a particular manufacturer's product should be based on clinical judgment and consultation with the patient and/or carer taking into account factors such as seizure frequency and treatment history.

Lacosamide

MHRA/CHM advice to minimize risk when switching patients with epilepsy between different manufacturers' products (incl. generic products):

- *Category 3*: it is usually unnecessary to ensure that patients are maintained on a specific manufacturer's product unless there are specific concerns, such as patient anxiety and risk of confusion/dosing error.

Indications

Rufinamide

Epilepsy: Adjunctive treatment of Lennox–Gastaut syndrome; refractory tonic/atonic seizures (unlicensed).

Lacosamide

Epilepsy: Adjunctive treatment of focal seizures with or without secondary generalization.

Perampanel

Epilepsy: Adjunctive treatment of focal seizures with or without secondary generalization and primary generalized tonic-clonic seizures.

Dose titration

Rufinamide

- *Epilepsy—adjunctive therapy (adults with body weight 30–50 kg)*: 200 mg bd for at least 2 days, then increased by 200 mg bd every 2 or more days (max. 900 mg bd).
- *Epilepsy—adjunctive therapy (adults with body weight 50–70 kg)*: 200 mg bd for at least 2 days, then increased by 200 mg bd every 2 or more days (max. 1200 mg bd).

- *Epilepsy—adjunctive therapy (adults with body weight above 70 kg)*: 200 mg bd for at least 2 days, then increased by 200 mg bd every 2 or more days (max. 1600 mg bd).

Lacosamide

- *Epilepsy—adjunctive therapy*: 50 mg bd for 7 days, then increased by 50 mg bd every 7 days; usual maintenance 100 mg bd (max. 200 mg bd).
- *Epilepsy—adjunctive therapy (loading dose regimen when it is necessary to rapidly attain therapeutic plasma concentrations, under close medical supervision)*: 200 mg bd for 1 day, followed by maintenance dose of 100 mg bd after 1 day, then increased if needed by 50 mg bd every 7 days (max. 200 mg bd).

Perampanel

Epilepsy—adjunctive therapy: 2 mg nocte for at least 14 days, then increased by 2 mg every 14 or more days; usual maintenance 4–8 mg nocte (max. 12 mg nocte).

Cautions

Rufinamide

Nil

Lacosamide

- Patients with conduction problems (contraindicated in patients with second- or third-degree A–V block).
- Patients with severe cardiac disease.
- Patients at risk of PR-interval prolongation.
- Elderly patients.

Perampanel

Nil

Adverse effects

Rufinamide

Rufinamide can be associated with adverse effects at the level the nervous system and other systems (Table 17.1).

Table 17.1 Estimated frequency of adverse effects of rufinamide

Very common (>1 in 10 patients on rufinamide)

Nervous system	Other systems
• dizziness • drowsiness • fatigue • headache	• nausea and vomiting

Common (>1 in 100 patients on rufinamide)

nervous system	Other systems
• anxiety • ataxia • blurred vision • convulsions • diplopia • gait disturbance • hyperactivity • insomnia • nystagmus • tremor	• dyspepsia, constipation, abdominal pain • acne • anorexia • back pain • diarrhoea • epistaxia • influenza-like symptoms • oligomenorrhoea • skin rash • rhinitis • weight loss

Uncommon (>1 in 1000 patients on rufinamide)

Nervous system	Other systems
	• Hypersensitivity syndromes including DRESS and Stevens–Johnson syndrome

Rare (>1 in 10,000 patients on rufinamide)

Nervous system	Other systems

Very rare (<1 in 10,000 patients on rufinamide)

Nervous system	Other systems

Lacosamide

Lacosamide can be associated with adverse effects at the level the nervous system and other systems (Table 17.2).

Table 17.2 Estimated frequency of adverse effects of lacosamide

Very common (>1 in 10 patients on lacosamide)	
Nervous system • diplopia • dizziness • headache	Other systems • nausea
Common (>1 in 100 patients on lacosamide)	
Nervous system • abnormal gait • amnesia • ataxia • blurred vision • confusion • depression • diplopia • drowsiness • fatigue • hypoaesthesia • irritability • nystagmus • tinnitus • tremor	Other systems • dry mouth • dyspepsia, constipation, flatulence • muscle spasms • pruritus • skin rash • vomiting
Uncommon (>1 in 1000 patients on lacosamide)	
Nervous system • aggression • agitation • psychosis • suicidal ideation	Other systems • atrial fibrillation, atrial flutter, AV block, PR interval prolongation • bradycardia
Rare (>1 in 10,000 patients on lacosamide)	
Nervous system	Other systems • multi-organ hypersensitivity reaction
Very rare (<1 in 10,000 patients on lacosamide)	
Nervous system	Other systems

Perampanel

Perampanel can be associated with adverse effects at the level the nervous system and other systems (Table 17.3).

Table 17.3 Estimated frequency of adverse effects of perampanel

Very common (>1 in 10 patients on perampanel)	
Nervous system • dizziness • drowsiness	Other systems

Common (>1 in 100 patients on perampanel)	
Nervous system • aggression • anxiety • ataxia • blurred vision • confusion • diplopia • dysarthria • gait disturbance • irritability • vertigo	Other systems • back pain • changes in appetite and weight gain • malaise • nausea

Uncommon (>1 in 1000 patients on perampanel)	
Nervous system • suicidal ideation and behaviour	Other systems

Rare (>1 in 10,000 patients on perampanel)	
Nervous system	Other systems

Very rare (<1 in 10,000 patients on perampanel)	
Nervous system	Other systems

Interactions

Rufinamide

With AEDs

Significant increases in rufinamide plasma concentrations may occur with co-administration of valproate.

With other drugs

- Women of child-bearing age using hormonal contraceptives are advised to use an additional safe and effective contraceptive method as co-administration of rufinamide has been shown to decrease exposure to a combined oral contraceptives.

- Rufinamide has been shown to induce the cytochrome P450 enzyme CYP3A4 and may, therefore, reduce the plasma concentrations of substances, which are metabolized by this enzyme (modest-to-moderate effect). It is therefore recommended that patients treated with substances that are metabolized by the CYP3A4 enzyme system are to be carefully monitored for 2 weeks at the start of or after the end of treatment with rufinamide, or after any marked change in the dose (a dose adjustment of the concomitantly administered medicinal product may need to be considered). These recommendations should also be considered when rufinamide is used concomitantly with substances with a narrow therapeutic window, such as warfarin and digoxin.

With alcohol/food

- No data on the interaction of rufinamide with alcohol are available
- As a food effect was observed, rufinamide should be administered with food

Lacosamide

With AEDs

Concomitant treatment with other AEDs known to be enzyme inducers (such as carbamazepine, phenobarbital, phenytoin) decreases the overall systemic exposure of lacosamide by 25%.

With other drugs

Nil.

With alcohol/food

- Although no pharmacokinetic data on the interaction of lacosamide with alcohol are available, a pharmacodynamic effect cannot be excluded.
- There are no specific foods that must be excluded from diet when taking lamotrigine.

Perampanel

With AEDs

- Some AEDs known as CYP450 3A enzyme inducers (carbamazepine, oxcarbazepine, phenytoin) have been shown to increase perampanel clearance and consequently to decrease plasma concentrations of perampanel. Carbamazepine, a known potent enzyme inducer, reduced perampanel levels by two-thirds in a study performed on healthy subjects
- In the epilepsy population pharmacokinetic analysis, perampanel was found to decrease the clearance of oxcarbazepine by 26%. Oxcarbazepine is rapidly metabolized by cytosolic reductase enzyme to the active

OTHER ANTIEPILEPTIC DRUGS • 143

metabolite, monohydroxycarbazepine. The effect of perampanel on monohydroxycarbazepine concentrations is not known

With other drugs

- Strong inducers of cytochrome P450, such as rifampicin and St John's wort (*Hypericum perforatum*), are expected to decrease perampanel concentrations.
- In healthy subjects, the CYP3A4 inhibitor ketoconazole increases perampanel exposure.
- Perampanel can make certain hormonal contraceptives such as levonorgestrel less effective.
- Decrease in exposure of midazolam may be caused by perampanel.

With alcohol/food

- Drinking alcohol while taking perampanel can affect a patients' alertness and ability to drive or use tools or machines. It can also aggravate irritability, confusion, and depression.
- There are no specific foods that must be excluded from diet when taking perampanel

Special populations

Rufinamide

Hepatic impairment

- Caution and careful dose titration in mild-to-moderate impairment
- Avoid in severe impairment

Renal impairment

The pharmacokinetics of rufinamide does not appear to be altered in subjects with chronic and severe renal failure compared to healthy volunteers

Pregnancy

- No clinical data are available on pregnancies exposed to rufinamide. Therefore, rufinamide should not be used during pregnancy or in women of childbearing age who are not using contraceptive measures, unless clearly necessary. Women of childbearing age must use contraceptive measures during treatment with rufinamide.
- If women treated with rufinamide plan to become pregnant, the continued use of this product should be carefully weighed. In case of treatment with rufinamide, the dose should be monitored carefully during pregnancy and after birth, and adjustments made on a clinical basis.

- It is not known if rufinamide is excreted in human breastmilk. Due to the potential harmful effects for the breastfed infant, breastfeeding should be avoided during maternal treatment with rufinamide.

Lacosamide

Hepatic impairment

- Titrate with caution in mild-to-moderate impairment if co-existing renal impairment.
- Caution in severe impairment.

Renal impairment

- Loading dose regimen can be considered in mild-to-moderate impairment (titrate above 200 mg with caution).
- Titrate with caution in severe impairment (max. 250 mg daily).

Pregnancy

- There are no adequate data from the use of lacosamide in pregnant women and the potential risk for humans is unknown.
- Lacosamide should not be used during pregnancy unless clearly necessary (if the benefit to the mother clearly outweighs the potential risk to the foetus). If a woman decides to become pregnant, the use of lacosamide should be carefully re-evaluated. In case of treatment with lacosamide, the dose should be monitored carefully during pregnancy and after birth, and adjustments made on a clinical basis.
- Lacosamide has been found to be present in milk in animal studies and it is recommended that it should be avoided during breastfeeding

Perampanel

Hepatic impairment

- Increase at intervals of at least 2 weeks, up to a maximum of 8 mg daily, in mild-to-moderate impairment.
- Avoid in severe impairment.

Renal impairment

Avoid in moderate or severe impairment.

Pregnancy

- There are limited amount of data available on the use of perampanel in pregnant women and the potential risk for humans is unknown.
- Perampanel is not recommended in pregnancy and female patients must use a reliable method of contraception to avoid becoming pregnant while

being treated with perampanel (this should be continued for 1 month after stopping treatment).
- As perampanel can make certain hormonal contraceptives such as levonorgestrel less effective, other forms of safe and effective contraception (such as a condom or coil) should be used when taking perampanel (this should be continued for 1 month after stopping treatment).
- Perampanel has been found to be present in milk in animal studies and it is recommended that breastfeeding should be avoided.

Behavioural and cognitive effects in patients with epilepsy

Rufinamide

For this third-generation agent, clinical experience is still limited, and little is known about its positive and negative psychotropic properties, and their implications for the management of behavioural symptoms in patients with epilepsy. There are initial reports of anxiety, depression, irritability, and agitation. Reports of cognitive effects are rare.

Lacosamide

For this third-generation agent, clinical experience is still limited and little is known about its positive and negative psychotropic properties and their implications for the management of behavioural symptoms in patients with epilepsy. There are initial reports of depression, irritability and agitation, and psychotic symptoms. Reports of cognitive effects (mainly affecting attention and memory) are rare and usually not severe.

Perampanel

For this third-generation agent, clinical experience is still limited, and little is known about its positive and negative psychotropic properties, and their implications for the management of behavioural symptoms in patients with epilepsy. There are initial reports of behavioural disturbances (especially depression, anxiety, irritability, and psychosis), which seem to be dose-related and tend to appear within the first weeks of treatment. Reports of cognitive effects (mainly affecting memory) are relatively rare.

Psychiatric use

Rufinamide

Rufinamide has no indications for the treatment of psychiatric disorders. There is insufficient experience with rufinamide to draw any conclusion regarding its psychotropic profile.

Lacosamide

Lacosamide has no indications for the treatment of psychiatric disorders. There is insufficient experience with lacosamide to draw any conclusion regarding its psychotropic profile.

Perampanel

Perampanel has no indications for the treatment of psychiatric disorders. There is insufficient experience with perampanel to draw any conclusion regarding its psychotropic profile.

CHAPTER 18

Comparative evidence and clinical scenarios

Behavioural profiles of antiepileptic drugs

The behavioural profiles of most antiepileptic drugs include both positive and negative effects, which can be usefully applied to clinical scenarios (Table 18.1).

Practical recommendations on the behavioural neurology of antiepileptic drugs

Based on the available evidence and clinical experience, it is possible to formulate a set of practical recommendations on the behavioural neurology of antiepileptic drugs (Table 18.2).

Psychiatric indications of antiepileptic drugs

Both clinical research and clinical experience support the use of antiepileptic drugs in patients with behavioural symptoms. Current evidence supporting the psychiatric use of antiepileptic drugs can be usefully summarized in a comparative chart (Fig. 18.1).

Table 18.1 Summary of the known behavioural profiles of antiepileptic drugs

AEDs	Positive effects			Negative effects		
	Antidepressant	Mood stabilizing	Anxiolythic	Depression	Irritability aggressiveness	Psychosis
Phenobarbital, primidone			+	+	+	
Phenytoin		+				+
Ethosuximide					+	+
Carbamazepine, oxcarbazepine		+				
Valproate		+	+			
Clonazepam, clobazam			+	+	+	
Vigabatrin				+	+	+
Lamotrigine	+	+			+	
Gabapentin			+		+	
Topiramate				+	+	+
Tiagabine				+	+	
Levetiracetam				+	+	+
Pregabalin			+	+	+	
Zonisamide				+	+	+

+ = Effect present.

Table 18.2 Summary of the practical recommendations on the behavioural neurology of antiepileptic drugs

AEDs	Depression	Bipolar disorder	Anxiety	Irritability	Psychosis	Substance abuse
Phenobarbital, primidone	−			−		
Phenytoin	−	+				
Ethosuximide					−	
Carbamazepine, oxcarbazepine		+		+		+
Valproate		+	+			+
Clonazepam, clobazam			+			
Vigabatrin	−			−	−	
Lamotrigine	+	+	−	−		+
Gabapentin			+	−		
Topiramate				−	−	
Tiagabine	−			−	−	
Levetiracetam	−		−	−	−	
Pregabalin			+			
Zonisamide					−	

+ = to consider (potential benefits); − = to avoid (alert).

150 • BEHAVIOURAL NEUROLOGY OF ANTIEPILEPTIC DRUGS

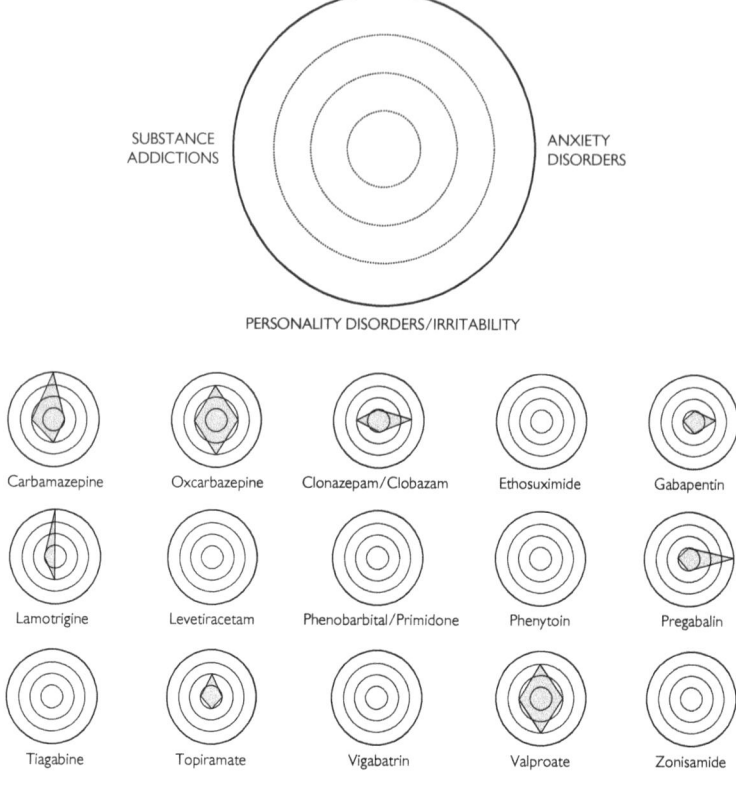

Fig. 18.1 Comparative chart of the level of evidence supporting the psychiatric use of antiepileptic drugs in patients with behavioural symptoms

References

BOOKS

Asadi-Pooya AA, Sperling MR. *Antiepileptic drugs: A clinician's manual*, 2nd edn. Oxford: Oxford University Press, 2016.

Ettinger AB, Kanner AM. *Psychiatric issues in epilepsy: A practical guide to diagnosis and treatment*, 2nd edn. Philadelphia, PA: Lippincott Williams & Wilkins, 2006.

Levy RH, Mattson RH, Meldrum BS, Perucca E (eds). *Antiepileptic drugs*, 5th edn. Philadelphia, PA: Lippincott Williams & Wilkins, 2002.

McElroy SL, Keck PE, Post RM (eds) *Antiepileptic drugs to treat psychiatric disorders*. New York, NY: Informa Healthcare USA, 2008.

Mula M (ed.) *Neuropsychiatric symptoms of epilepsy*. Heidelberg: Springer, 2016.

National Institute for Health and Care Excellence (NICE). Clinical Guideline (CG137) *Epilepsies: Diagnosis and Management*. NICE, 2012 (updated 2016).

Panayiotopoulos CP (ed.) *Atlas of epilepsies*. London: Springer, 2010.

Patsalos PN. *Antiepileptic drug interactions: A clinical guide*, 2nd edn. London: Springer, 2013.

Patsalos PN, Bourgeois BFD. *The epilepsy prescriber's guide to antiepileptic drugs*, 2nd edn. Cambridge: Cambridge University Press, 2013.

Pohlmann-Eden B, Steinhoff BJ. *Understanding antiepileptic drugs: Guiding you through the maze of options*. Oxford: Oxford University Press, 2014.

Schachter SC, Holmes GL, Kasteleijn-Nolst Trenité (eds) *Behavioral aspects of epilepsy: Principles and practice*. New York, NY: Demos, 2008.

Shorvon SD. *Handbook of epilepsy treatment*, 3rd edn. Oxford: Wiley-Blackwell 2010.

Shorvon SD, Perucca E, Engel J Jr (eds) *The treatment of epilepsy*, 4th edn. Oxford: Wiley-Blackwell, 2015.

Silberstein SD, Marmura MJ, Yuan H. *Essential neuropharmacology: Prescriber's guide*, 2nd edn. Cambridge: Cambridge University Press, 2015.

Stahl SM. *Stahl's essential psychopharmacology: Neuroscientific basis and practical applications*, 4th edn. Cambridge: Cambridge University Press, 2013.

Stahl SM. *Stahl's essential psychopharmacology: Prescriber' guide*, 5th edn. Cambridge: Cambridge University Press, 2014.

Trimble MR, Schmitz B (eds) *Forced normalization and alternative psychoses of epilepsy*. Petersfield: Wrightson Biomedical Publishing, 1998.

Trimble MR, Schmitz B (eds) *Seizures, affective disorders and anticonvulsant drugs*. Guildford: Clarius Press, 2002.

Trimble MR, Schmitz B (eds) *The neuropsychiatry of epilepsy*, 2nd edn. Cambridge: Cambridge University Press, 2011.

Wyllie E (ed.) *Wyllie's treatment of epilepsy: Principles and practice*, 5th edn. Philadelphia, PA: Lippincott Williams & Wilkins, 2011.

BOOK CHAPTERS

Kaufman KR. Antiepileptic drugs in the treatment of psychiatric disorders. In: Panayiotopoulos CP (ed.) *Atlas of epilepsies*. London: Springer, 2010, pp. 1571–6.

Schmitz B. The effects of antiepileptic drugs on behaviour. In: Trimble MR, Schmitz B (eds) *The neuropsychiatry of epilepsy*, 2nd edn. Cambridge: Cambridge University Press, 2011, pp. 133–42.

Yogarajah M, Mula M. The role of antiepileptic drugs. In: Mula M (ed.) *Neuropsychiatric symptoms of epilepsy*. Heidelberg: Springer, 2016, pp. 333–60.

ARTICLES

Ali F, Rickards H, Cavanna AE. The assessment of consciousness during partial seizures. *Epilepsy and Behavior* 2012; **23**: 98–102.

Baldwin DS, den Boer JA, Lyndon G, Emir B, Schweizer E, Haswell H. Efficacy and safety of pregabalin in generalised anxiety disorder: A critical review of the literature. *Journal of Psychopharmacology* 2015; **29**: 1047–60.

Bangar S, Shastri A, El-Sayeh H, Cavanna AE. Women with epilepsy: Clinically relevant issues. *Functional Neurology* 2016; **31**: 127–34.

Berg AT, Altalib HH, Devinsky O. Psychiatric and behavioral comorbidities in epilepsy: A critical reappraisal. *Epilepsia* 2017; **58**: 1123–30.

Berlin RK, Butler PM, Perloff MD. Gabapentin therapy in psychiatric disorders: A systematic review. *Primary Care Companion for CNS Disorders* 2015; **17**: 5.

Besag FM, Patsalos PN. Clinical efficacy of perampanel for partial-onset and primary generalized tonic-clonic seizures. *Neuropsychiatric Disease and Treatment* 2016; **12**: 1215–20.

Bialer M. Why are antiepileptic drugs used for nonepileptic conditions? *Epilepsia* 2012; **53**(Suppl. 7): 26–33.

Blumer D. Evidence supporting the temporal lobe epilepsy personality syndrome. *Neurology* 1999; **53**(Suppl. 2): 9–12.

Boylan LS, Devinsky O, Barry JJ, Ketter TA. Psychiatric uses of antiepileptic treatments. *Epilepsy & Behavior* 2002; **3**: 54–9.

Brandt C, Mula M. Anxiety disorders in people with epilepsy. *Epilepsy & Behavior* 2016; **59**: 87–91.

Brodie MJ. Antiepileptic drug therapy: The story so far. *Seizure* 2010; **19**: 650–5.

Brodie MJ, Besag F, Ettinger AB, Mula M, Gobbi G, Comai S, Aldenkamp AP, Steinhoff BJ. Epilepsy, antiepileptic drugs, and aggression: An evidence-based review. *Pharmacological Reviews* 2016; **68**: 563–602.

Brodtkorb E, Mula M. Optimizing therapy of seizures in adult patients with psychiatric comorbidity. *Neurology* 2006; **67**(Suppl. 4): 39–44.

Brunbech L, Sabers A. Effect of antiepileptic drugs on cognitive function in individuals with epilepsy: A comparative review of newer versus older agents. *Drugs* 2002; **62**: 593–604.

Buoli M, Grassi S, Ciappolino V, Serati M, Altamura AC. The use of zonisamide for the treatment of psychiatric disorders: A systematic review. *Clinical Neuropharmacology* 2017; **40**: 85–92.

Caputo F, Bernardi M. Medications acting on the GABA system in the treatment of alcoholic patients. *Current Pharmaceutical Design* 2010; **16**: 2118–25.

Cavanna AE. Epilepsy, behavior, and neuropsychiatry. *Epilepsy & Behavior* 2014; **40**: 78.

Cavanna AE, Ali F, Rickards HE, McCorry D. Behavioural and cognitive effects of antiepileptic drugs. *Discovery Medicine* 2010; **9**: 138–44.

Cavanna AE, Cavanna S, Bertero L, Robertson MM. Depression in women with epilepsy: Clinical and neurobiological aspects. *Functional Neurology* 2009; **24**: 83–7.

Cavanna AE, Rickards H, Ali F. What makes a simple partial seizure complex? *Epilepsy and Behavior* 2011; **22**: 651–8.

Cavanna AE, Seri S. Psychiatric adverse effects of Zonisamide in patients with epilepsy and mental disorder comorbidities. *Epilepsy & Behavior* 2013; **29**: 281–4.

Cipriani A, Reid K, Young AH, Macritchie K, Geddes J. Valproic acid, valproate and divalproex in the maintenance treatment of bipolar disorder. *Cochrane Database of Systematic Reviews* 2013; **10**: CD003196.

Cox JH, Seri S, Cavanna AE. Zonisamide as a treatment for partial epileptic seizures: A systematic review. *Advances in Therapy* 2014; **31**: 276–88.

Devinsky O. Cognitive and behavioral effects of antiepileptic drugs. *Epilepsia* 1995; **36**(Suppl. 2): 46–65.

Devinsky O, Najjar S. Evidence against the existence of a temporal lobe epilepsy personality syndrome. *Neurology* 1999; **53**(Suppl. 2): 13–25.

D'Souza J, Johnson M, Borghs S. Meta-analysis of nonpsychotic behavioral treatment emergent adverse events in brivaracetam and levetiracetam development programs. *Epilepsia* 2012; **53**(Suppl. 5): 118.

Eddy CM, Rickards H, Cavanna AE. Behavioral adverse effects of antiepileptic drugs in epilepsy. *Journal of Clinical Psychopharmacology* 2012; **32**: 362–75.

Eddy CM, Rickards HE, Cavanna AE. The cognitive impact of antiepileptic drugs. *Therapeutic Advances in Neurological Disorders* 2011; **4**: 380–402.

Ettinger AB. Antiepileptics for psychiatric illness: Find the right match. *Current Psychiatry* 2010; **9**: 50–66.

Ettinger AB. Psychotropic effects of antiepileptic drugs. *Neurology* 2006; **67**: 1916–25.

Frampton JE. Pregabalin: A review of its use in adults with generalized anxiety disorder. *CNS Drugs* 2014; **28**: 835–54.

Generoso MB, Trevizol AP, Kasper S, Cho HJ, Cordeiro Q, Shiozawa P. Pregabalin for generalized anxiety disorder: An updated systematic review and meta-analysis. *International Clinical Psychopharmacology* 2017; **32**: 49–55.

Gilliam FG, Barry JJ, Hermann BP, Meador KJ, Vahle V, Kanner AM. Rapid detection of major depression in epilepsy: A multicenter study. *Lancet Neurology* 2006; **5**: 399–405.

Golyala A, Kwan P. Drug development for refractory epilepsy: The past 25 years and beyond. *Seizure* 2017; **44**: 147–56.

Grunze HC. Anticonvulsants in bipolar disorder. *Journal of Mental Health* 2010; **19**: 127–41.

Guglielmo R, Martinotti G, Clerici M, Janiri L. Pregabalin for alcohol dependence: A critical review of the literature. *Advances in Therapy* 2012; **29**: 947–57.

Guglielmo R, Martinotti G, Quatrale M, Ioime L, Kadilli I, Di Nicola M, Janiri L. Topiramate in alcohol use disorders: Review and update. *CNS Drugs* 2015; **29**: 383–95.

Hermann B, Meador KJ, Gaillard WD, Cramer JA. Cognition across the lifespan: Antiepileptic drugs, epilepsy, or both? *Epilepsy & Behavior* 2010; **17**: 1–5.

Jerath NU, Lamichhane D, Jasti M, et al. Treating epilepsy in the setting of medical comorbidities. *Current Treatment Options in Neurology* 2014; **16**: 298.

Johannessen Landmark C. Antiepileptic drugs in non-epilepsy disorders: Relations between mechanisms of action and clinical efficacy. *CNS Drugs* 2008; **22**: 27–47.

Johnson BA, Ait-Daoud N. Topiramate in the new generation of drugs: Efficacy in the treatment of alcoholic patients. *Current Pharmaceutical Design* 2010; **16**:2103–12.

Jones R, Rickards H, Cavanna AE. The prevalence of psychiatric disorders in epilepsy: A critical review of the evidence. *Functional Neurology* 2010; **25**: 191–4.

Jones RM, Arlidge J, Gillham R, Reagu S, van den Bree M, Taylor PJ. Efficacy of mood stabilisers in the treatment of impulsive or repetitive aggression: Systematic review and meta-analysis. *British Journal of Psychiatry* 2011; **198**: 93–8.

Kanner AM. Management of psychiatric and neurological comorbidities in epilepsy. *Nature Reviews Neurology* 2016; **12**: 106–16.

Kanner AM. Psychiatric comorbidities in new onset epilepsy: Should they be always investigated? *Seizure* 2017; **49**: 79–82.

Kanner AM, Palac S. Neuropsychiatric complications of epilepsy. *Current Neurology and Neuroscience Reports* 2002; **2**: 365–72.

Kaufman KR. Antiepileptic drugs in the treatment of psychiatric disorders. *Epilepsy & Behavior* 2011; **21**: 1–11.

Kaufman KR. Use of antiepileptic drugs for nonepileptic conditions: Psychiatric disorders and chronic pain. *Neurotherapeutics* 2007; **4**: 75–83.

Kerr MP, Mensah S, Besag F, et al. International consensus clinical practice statements for the treatment of neuropsychiatric conditions associated with epilepsy. *Epilepsia* 2011; **52**: 2133–8.

Ketter TA, Post RM, Theodore WH. Positive and negative psychiatric effects of antiepileptic drugs in patients with seizure disorders. *Neurology* 1999; **53**(Suppl. 2): 53–67.

Kimiskidis VK, Valeta T. Epilepsy and anxiety: Epidemiology, classification, aetiology, and treatment. *Epileptic Disorders* 2012; **14**: 248–56.

Kinrys G, Worthington JJ, Wygant L, Nery F, Reese H, Pollack MH. Levetiracetam as adjunctive therapy for refractory anxiety disorders. *Journal of Clinical Psychiatry* 2007; **68**: 1010–13.

Kirmani BF, Robinson DM, Kikam A, Fonkem E, Cruz D. Selection of antiepileptic drugs in older people. *Current Treatment Options in Neurology* 2014; **16**: 295.

Krasowski MD. Therapeutic drug monitoring of the newer anti-epilepsy medications. *Pharmaceuticals* 2010; **3**: 1909–35.

Krishnamoorthy ES. The evaluation of behavioral disturbances in epilepsy. *Epilepsia* 2006; **47**(Suppl. 2): 3–8.

Krishnamoorthy ES, Trimble MR, Blumer D. The classification of neuropsychiatric disorders in epilepsy: A proposal by the ILAE Commission on Psychobiology of Epilepsy. *Epilepsy & Behavior* 2007; **10**: 349–53.

Langan J, Perry A, Oto M. Teratogenic risk and contraceptive counselling in psychiatric practice: Analysis of anticonvulsant therapy. *BMC Psychiatry* 2013; **13**: 234.

Lennox WG, Markham CH. The socio-psychological treatment of epilepsy. *Journal of the American Medical Association* 1953; **152**: 1690–4.

Lin JJ, Mula M, Hermann BP. Uncovering the neurobehavioural comorbidities of epilepsy over the lifespan. *Lancet* 2012; **380**: 1180–92.

Loganathan MA, Enja M, Lippmann S. Forced normalization: Epilepsy and psychosis interaction. *Innovations in Clinical Neuroscience* 2015; **12**: 38–41.

López-Muñoz F, Ucha-Udabe R, Alamo C. The history of barbiturates a century after their clinical introduction. *Neuropsychiatric Disease and Treatment* 2005; **1**: 329–43.

Luykx JJ, Carpay JA. Nervous system adverse responses to topiramate in the treatment of neuropsychiatric disorders. *Expert Opinion on Drug Safety* 2010; **9**: 623–31.

Malykh AG, Sadaie MR. Piracetam and piracetam-like drugs: From basic science to novel clinical applications to CNS disorders. *Drugs* 2010; **70**: 287–312.

Maremmani I, Pacini M, Lamanna F, et al. Mood stabilizers in the treatment of substance use disorders. *CNS Spectrums* 2010; **15**: 95–109.

Mariani JJ, Levin FR. Levetiracetam for the treatment of co-occurring alcohol dependence and anxiety: Case series and review. *American Journal of Drug and Alcohol Abuse* 2008; **34**: 683–91.

Martin K, Katz A. The role of barbiturates for alcohol withdrawal syndrome. *Psychosomatics* 2016; **57**: 341–7.

Martinotti G, Lupi M, Sarchione F, et al. The potential of pregabalin in neurology, psychiatry and addiction: A qualitative overview. *Current Pharmaceutical Design* 2013; **19**: 6367–74.

McIntyre RS, Cha DS, Kim RD, Mansur RB. A review of FDA-approved treatment options in bipolar depression. *CNS Spectrums* 2013; **18**(Suppl. 1): 4–20.

Meador KJ, Gilliam FG, Kanner AM, Pellock JM. Cognitive and behavioral effects of antiepileptic drugs. *Epilepsy & Behavior* 2001; **2**(Suppl.): 1–17.

Mersfelder TL, Nichols WH. Gabapentin: Abuse, dependence, and withdrawal. *Annals of Pharmacotherapy* 2016; **50**: 229–33.

Mitchell JW, Seri S, Cavanna AE. Pharmacotherapeutic options for refractory and difficult-to-treat seizures. *Journal of Central Nervous System Disease* 2012; **4**: 105–15.

Miura T, Noma H, Furukawa TA, et al. Comparative efficacy and tolerability of pharmacological treatments in the maintenance treatment of bipolar disorder: A systematic review and network meta-analysis. *Lancet Psychiatry* 2014; **1**: 351–9.

Motamedi GK, Meador KJ. Antiepileptic drugs and memory. *Epilepsy & Behavior* 2004; **5**: 435–9.

Motamedi GK, Meador KJ. Epilepsy and cognition. *Epilepsy & Behavior* 2003; **4**(Suppl.): 25–38.

Mula M. Epilepsy and psychiatric comorbidities: Drug selection. *Current Treatment Options in Neurology* 2017; **19**: 44.

Mula M. Investigating psychotropic properties of antiepileptic drugs. *Expert Review of Neurotherapeutics* 2013; **13**: 639–46.

Mula M. Recent and future antiepileptic drugs and their impact on cognition: what can we expect? *Expert Reviews of Neurotherapeutics* 2012; **12**: 667–71.

Mula M. The interictal dysphoric disorder of epilepsy: Legend or reality? *Epilepsy & Behavior* 2016; **58**: 7–10.

Mula M, Cavanna AE, Monaco F. Psychopharmacology of topiramate: From epilepsy to bipolar disorder. *Neuropsychiatric Disease and Treatment* 2006; **2**: 475–88.

Mula M, Kanner AM, Schmitz B, Schachter S. Antiepileptic drugs and suicidality: An expert consensus statement from the Task Force on Therapeutic Strategies of the ILAE Commission on Neuropsychobiology. *Epilepsia* 2013; **54**: 199–203.

Mula M, Pini S, Cassano GB. The role of anticonvulsant drugs in anxiety disorders: A critical review of the evidence. *Journal of Clinical Psychopharmacology* 2007; **27**: 263–72.

Mula M, Sander JW. Negative effects of antiepileptic drugs on mood in patients with epilepsy. *Drug Safety* 2007; **30**: 555–67.

Nadkarni S, Arnedo V, Devinsky O. Psychosis in epilepsy patients. *Epilepsia* 2007; **48**(Suppl. 9): 17–19.

Nadkarni S, Devinsky O. Psychotropic effects of antiepileptic drugs. *Epilepsy Currents* 2005; **5**: 176–81.

Nardi AE, Machado S, Almada LF, et al. Clonazepam for the treatment of panic disorder. *Current Drug Targets* 2013; **14**: 353–64.

Nardi AE, Perna G. Clonazepam in the treatment of psychiatric disorders: An update. *International Clinical Psychopharmacology* 2006; **21**: 131–42.

Nogueira MH, Yasuda CL, Coan AC, Kanner AM, Cendes F. Concurrent mood and anxiety disorders are associated with pharmacoresistant seizures in patients with MTLE. *Epilepsia* 2017; **58**: 1268–76.

Ortinski P, Meador KJ. Cognitive side effects of antiepileptic drugs. *Epilepsy & Behavior* 2004; **5**(Suppl.): 60–5.

Osman A, Seri S, Cavanna AE. Clinical characteristics of patients with epilepsy in a specialist neuropsychiatry service. *Epilepsy & Behavior* 2016; **58**: 44–7.

Oulis P, Konstantakopoulos G. Efficacy and safety of pregabalin in the treatment of alcohol and benzodiazepine dependence. *Expert Opinion on Investigational Drugs* 2012; **21**: 1019–29.

Pacchiarotti I, León-Caballero J, Murru A, et al. Mood stabilizers and antipsychotics during breastfeeding: Focus on bipolar disorder. *European Neuropsychopharmacology* 2016; **26**: 1562–78.

Perucca P, Carter J, Vahle V, Gilliam FG. Adverse antiepileptic drug effects: Toward a clinically and neurobiologically relevant taxonomy. *Neurology* 2009; **72**: 1223–9.

Perucca P, Gilliam FG. Adverse effects of antiepileptic drugs. *Lancet Neurology* 2012; **11**: 792–802.

Perucca P, Mula M. Antiepileptic drug effects on mood and behavior: Molecular targets. *Epilepsy & Behavior* 2013; **26**: 440–9.

Pichler EM, Hattwich G, Grunze H, Muehlbacher M. Safety and tolerability of anticonvulsant medication in bipolar disorder. *Expert Opinion on Drug Safety* 2015; **14**: 1703–24.

Piedad J, Rickards H, Besag F, Cavanna AE. Beneficial and adverse psychotropic effects of antiepileptic drugs in patients with epilepsy: A summary of prevalence, underlying mechanisms and data limitations. *CNS Drugs* 2012; **26**: 319–35.

Pigott K, Galizia I, Vasudev K, Watson S, Geddes J, Young AH. Topiramate for acute affective episodes in bipolar disorder in adults. *Cochrane Database of Systematic Reviews* 2016; **9**: CD003384.

Reid JG, Gitlin MJ, Altshuler LL. Lamotrigine in psychiatric disorders. *Journal of Clinical Psychiatry* 2013; **74**: 675–84.

Rogawski MA, Löscher W. The neurobiology of antiepileptic drugs for the treatment of nonepileptic conditions. *Nature Medicine* 2004; **10**: 685–92.

Ruiz-Giménez J, Sánchez-Alvarez JC, Cañadillas-Hidalgo F, Serrano-Castro PJ, Andalusian Epilepsy Society. Antiepileptic treatment in patients with epilepsy and other comorbidities. *Seizure* 2010; **19**: 375–82.

Santulli L, Coppola A, Balestrini S, Striano S. The challenges of treating epilepsy with 25 antiepileptic drugs. *Pharmacological Research* 2016; **107**: 211–19.

Schmitz B. Effects of antiepileptic drugs on mood and behavior. *Epilepsia* 2006; **47**(Suppl. 2): 28–33.

Schmitz B. Psychiatric syndromes related to antiepileptic drugs. *Epilepsia* 1999; **40**(Suppl. 10): 65–70.

Schwartz TL, Nihalani N. Tiagabine in anxiety disorders. *Expert Opinion on Pharmacotherapy* 2006; **7**: 1977–87.

Scott DF. The discovery of anti-epileptic drugs. *Journal of the History of the Neurosciences* 1992; **1**: 111–18.

Shinn AK, Greenfield SF. Topiramate in the treatment of substance-related disorders: A critical review of the literature. *Journal of Clinical Psychiatry* 2010; **71**: 634–48.

Shorvon SD. Drug treatment of epilepsy in the century of the ILAE: The first 50 years, 1909–1958. *Epilepsia* 2009; **50**(Suppl. 3): 69–92.

Shorvon SD. Drug treatment of epilepsy in the century of the ILAE: The second 50 years, 1959–2009. *Epilepsia* 2009; **50**(Suppl. 3): 93–130.

Singh M, Keer D, Klimas J, Wood E, Werb D. Topiramate for cocaine dependence: A systematic review and meta-analysis of randomized controlled trials. *Addiction* 2016; **111**: 1337–46.

Siniscalchi A, Gallelli L, Russo E, De Sarro G. A review on antiepileptic drugs-dependent fatigue: Pathophysiological mechanisms and incidence. *European Journal of Pharmacology* 2013; **718**: 10–16.

Spina E, Perugi G. Antiepileptic drugs: Indications other than epilepsy. *Epileptic Disorders* 2004; **6**: 57–75.

Spitzer RL, Kroenke K, Williams JBW, Lowe B. A brief measure for assessing generalized anxiety disorder. *Archives of Internal Medicine* 2006; **166**: 1092–7.

Stahl SM, Porreca F, Taylor CP, Cheung R, Thorpe AJ, Clair A. The diverse therapeutic actions of pregabalin: is a single mechanism responsible for several pharmacological activities? *Trends in Pharmacological Sciences* 2013; **34**: 332–9.

Tomson T, Battino D. Teratogenic effects of antiepileptic drugs. *Lancet Neurology* 2012; **11**: 803–13.

Uguz F, Sharma V. Mood stabilizers during breastfeeding: A systematic review of the recent literature. *Bipolar Disorders* 2016; **18**: 325–33.

Vajda FJ, Dodd S, Horgan D. Lamotrigine in epilepsy, pregnancy and psychiatry: a drug for all seasons? *Journal of Clinical Neurosciences* 2013; **20**: 13–16.

Vajda FJE, Eadie MJ. Perucca P, Mula M. The clinical pharmacology of traditional antiepileptic drugs. *Epileptic Disorders* 2014; **16**: 395–408.

Vasudev A, Macritchie K, Rao SK, Geddes J, Young AH. Tiagabine for acute affective episodes in bipolar disorder. *Cochrane Database of Systematic Reviews* 2012; **12**: CD004694.

Vasudev A, Macritchie K, Rao SN, Geddes J, Young AH. Tiagabine in the maintenance treatment of bipolar disorder. *Cochrane Database of Systematic Reviews* 2011; **12**: CD005173.

Vasudev A, Macritchie K, Vasudev K, Watson S, Geddes J, Young AH. Oxcarbazepine for acute affective episodes in bipolar disorder. *Cochrane Database of Systematic Reviews* 2011; **12**: CD004857.

Vigo DV, Baldessarini RJ. Anticonvulsants in the treatment of major depressive disorder: An overview. *Harvard Review of Psychiatry* 2009; **17**: 231–41.

Villari V, Rocca P, Frieri T, Bogetto F. Psychiatric symptoms related to the use of lamotrigine: A review of the literature. *Functional Neurology* 2008; **23**: 133–6.

Wang HR, Woo YS, Bahk WM. Potential role of anticonvulsants in the treatment of obsessive-compulsive and related disorders. *Psychiatry and Clinical Neurosciences* 2014; **68**: 723–32.

Williams JW Jr, Ranney L, Morgan LC, Whitener L. How reviews covered the unfolding scientific story of gabapentin for bipolar disorder. *General Hospital Psychiatry* 2009; **31**: 279–87.

Witt J-A, Helmstaedter C. Monitoring the cognitive effects of antiepileptic pharmacotherapy: Approaching the individual patient. *Epilepsy & Behavior* 2013; **26**: 450–6.

Yasiry Z, Shorvon SD. How phenobarbital revolutionized epilepsy therapy: The story of phenobarbital therapy in epilepsy in the last 100 years. *Epilepsia* 2012; **53**(Suppl. 8): 26–39.

Zaccara G, Perucca E. Interactions between antiepileptic drugs, and between antiepileptic drugs and other drugs. *Epileptic Disorders* 2014; **16**: 409–31.

Zhuo C, Jiang R, Li G, et al. Efficacy and tolerability of second and third generation antiepileptic drugs in refractory epilepsy: A network meta-analysis. *Scientific Reports* 2017; **7**: 2535.

Index

NOTE: *f* denotes figure, and *t* table

A

affective disorders 3–5
aggressiveness, effects of AEDs 148*t*
antidepressant effects of AEDS 148*t*
antiepileptic drugs (AEDs) 7–20
 chronology of clinical use 10*f*
 first-, second-, third-generation 7, 21
 mechanisms of action 8*t*
 psychiatric use, indications (all AEDs) 148*t*
  comparative chart, level of evidence 150*f*
 psychotropic effects 3
anxiety disorders 3–5, 36, 38, 46, 47, 56, 60, 74, 128
 effects of AEDs 148–9*t*
 see also psychiatric use
Aptiom® *see* eslicarbazepine
atrioventricular block 26, 29

B

Banzel® *see* rufinamide
behavioural neurology
 co-morbidities in epilepsy 1–6
 early recognition and initial evaluation 3
 practical recommendations (all AEDs) 149*t*
 profiles (all AEDs) 148*t*, 150*f*
bipolar disorder (mania) 24–5, 36, 37, 47, 53, 67, 117, 121, 125*t*
 effects of AEDs 149*t*
bone marrow depression 26, 31
brivaracetam 7, 9*t*, 19, 75–6
Briviact® *see* brivaracetam

C

carbamazepine 7, 8*t*, 12, 21–38
 behavioural/cognitive effects in epilepsy 35–6
 cautions, adverse effects 26–8*t*, 50–1*t*
 dose titration 25
 generic formulation 23
 indications 24
 interactions
  with AEDs 31
  with alcohol/food 32
  with other drugs 31–2
 overall rating 38*t*
 plasma levels monitoring 25–6
 pregnancy; hepatic and renal impairment 33–4
 preparations and structure 21–3*f*
 psychiatric use 36–7*f*
 related AEDs 7, 8*t*, 21
cardiac disease 26, 138
clobazam 7, 8*t*, 14, 39–48
 adverse effects 44*t*
 behavioural/cognitive effects in epilepsy 46
 dose titration 42
 generic formulation 41
 indications 41
 interactions
  with AEDs 45
  with alcohol/food 45
  with other drugs 45
 overall rating 47*t*
 pregnancy; hepatic and renal impairment 45–6
 preparations and structure 39–40*f*
 psychiatric use 47*f*
 recommendations from NICE 41
clonazepam 7, 8*t*, 13, 39–48
 adverse effects 42, 43*t*
 behavioural/cognitive effects in epilepsy 46
 cautions 42
 dose titration 41
 generic formulation 41
 indications 41
 interactions
  with AEDs 43
  with alcohol/food 44
  with other drugs 43
 overall rating 47*t*
 plasma levels monitoring 42
 pregnancy; hepatic and renal impairment 45
 preparations and structure 39–40*f*
 psychiatric use 46–7*f*
 recommendations from NICE 41
comparative chart, level of evidence for psychiatric use (all AEDs) 148–9*t*
coordination, impaired 110

D

Depakote® *see* valproate
depression, effects of AEDS 148–9*t*
Dilantin® *see* phenytoin
diplopia 27, 29, 30, 65, 72, 96, 125, 131, 139, 140, 141
Dravet syndrome 24, 25, 56, 62, 86, 94, 101, 117, 124

E

Epanutin® *see* phentoiny
Epilim® *see* valproate
Episenta® *see* valproate
eslicarbazepine 7, 9*t*, 18–19, 21–38
 adverse effects 30*t*
 behavioural/cognitive effects in epilepsy 36
 cautions 26
 dose titration 25
 generic formulation 24
 indications 25
 interactions
  with AEDs 33
  with alcohol/food 33
  with other drugs 33
 overall rating 39
 plasma levels monitoring 26
 pregnancy; hepatic and renal impairment 35
 preparations and structure 23*f*
 psychiatric use 38
 recommendations from NICE 25
ethosuximide 7, 8*t*, 12, 49–53
 behavioural/cognitive effects in epilepsy 52–3*f*
 cautions, adverse effects 50–1*t*
 dose titration 50
 generic formulation 50
 indications 50
 interactions
  with AEDs 51–2
  with alcohol/food 52
  with other drugs 52
 overall rating 53*t*
 plasma levels monitoring 25–6
 pregnancy; hepatic and renal impairment 52
 preparations and structure 49*f*
 psychiatric use 53*f*
 recommendations from NICE 50
excluded agents *viii*

F

Fycompa® *see* perampanel

G

gabapentin 7, 8*t*, 15–16, 55–60
 behavioural/cognitive effects in epilepsy 59
 cautions, adverse effects 57, 58*t*
 dose titration 57

160 • INDEX

gabapentin (cont.)
  generic formulation 55
  indications 55
  interactions
    with AEDs 57
    with alcohol/food 59
    with other drugs 57
  overall rating 60t
  plasma levels monitoring 57
  preparations and
    structure 55–6f
  psychiatric use 59–60f
  recommendations from
    NICE 56–7
Gabitril® see tiagabine
Gastaut–Geschwind syndrome 2
glaucoma 26, 28, 111

H

hallucinations 4, 5, 27, 52, 65, 80, 81, 96, 132
hearing disorders 28
HLA-B*1502 28, 29, 88
hyponatraemia 26, 27, 29, 30, 118

I

impaired coordination 110
Invelon® see rufinamide
irritability, effects of
  AEDs 148t, 149t

K

Keppra® see levetiracetam

L

lacosamide 7, 9t, 20, 135–46
  behavioural/cognitive effects in
    epilepsy 145
  cautions, adverse
    effects 139–40t
  dose titration 138
  generic formulation 137
  indications 137
  interactions
    with AEDs 142
    with alcohol/food 142
  pregnancy; hepatic and renal
    impairment 144
  preparations and structure 136f
  psychiatric use 146
Lamictal® see lamotrigine
lamotrigine 7, 8t, 15, 61–8
  behavioural/cognitive effects in
    epilepsy 66
  cautions, adverse effects 58t, 64
  dose titration 63
  interactions
    with AEDs 64
    with alcohol/food 66
    with other drugs 64
  overall rating 68t
  plasma levels monitoring 64
  pregnancy; hepatic and renal
    impairment 66

preparations and
    structure 61–2f
  psychiatric use 67f
  recommendations from
    NICE 62
Lennox–Gastaut syndrome 19, 24, 25, 56, 62, 94, 101, 108, 117, 124, 137
levetiracetam 7, 8t, 17, 69–74
  adverse effects 71–2t
  behavioural/cognitive effects in
    epilepsy 73
  dose titration 71
  interactions
    with alcohol/food 72
    with other drugs 71
  overall rating 74t
  plasma levels monitoring 71
  pregnancy; hepatic and renal
    impairment 71
  preparations and
    structure 69–70f
  psychiatric use 73–4f
  recommendations from
    NICE 70
Lyrica® see pregabalin

M

mania, acute 24, 25, 36, 37, 47, 53, 117, 121, 125t
metabolic acidosis 109, 110, 131, 132
mood stabilizing effects of
  AEDs 148–9t

N

nephrolithiasis 109, 131
Neurontin® see gabapentin
Nootropil® see piracetam
nystagmus 27, 29, 30, 43, 58, 65, 80, 81, 118, 125, 131, 139, 140

O

obsessive–compulsive
  disorder 38, 42, 113
oxcarbazepine 7, 8t, 17, 21–38
  adverse effects 29t
  behavioural/cognitive effects in
    epilepsy 35
  cautions 26
  dose titration 25
  generic formulation 24
  indications 24
  interactions
    with AEDs 32
    with alcohol/food 32
    with other drugs 32
  overall rating 38t
  plasma levels monitoring 26
  pregnancy; hepatic and renal
    impairment 34–5, 59
  preparations and structure 22–3f
  psychiatric use 37f
  recommendations from
    NICE 24

P

Panayiotopoulos syndrome 24, 25, 56, 62, 70, 79, 86, 94, 101, 108, 117, 124, 130
perampanel 7, 9t, 20, 135–46
  adverse effects 141t
  behavioural/cognitive effects in
    epilepsy 145
  dose titration 138
  generic formulation 137
  indications 137
  interactions
    with AEDs 142
    with alcohol/food 143
    with other drugs 143
  pregnancy; hepatic and renal
    impairment 144
  preparations and
    structure 136f
  psychiatric use 146
personality disorders, levels of
  evidence 47, 53, 60, 67, 74, 83, 91, 98, 105, 122, 127, 134, 150f
phenobarbital 7, 8t, 10, 77–84
  adverse effects 79–80t
  behavioural/cognitive effects in
    epilepsy 83–4
  chronology of clinical use 78f
  dose titration 79
  interactions
    with AEDs 80–1
    with alcohol/food 82
    with other drugs 82
  overall rating 84
  plasma levels monitoring 79
  pregnancy; hepatic and renal
    impairment 82–3
  preparations and
    structure 77–8f
  psychiatric use 83f, 84
  recommendations from
    NICE 79
phenytoin 7, 8t, 11, 85–92
  adverse effects 88t
  behavioural/cognitive effects in
    epilepsy 90
  dose titration 87
  generic formulation 85
  indications 86
  interactions
    with AEDs 87
    with alcohol/food 89
    with other drugs 88
  overall rating 91
  plasma levels monitoring 87
  pregnancy; hepatic and renal
    impairment 90
  preparations and
    structure 85–6f
  psychiatric use 90–1f
  recommendations from
    NICE 86
phobias 3, 46, 60, 110
photophobia 51, 110
piracetam 7, 8t, 14, 75
porphyrias 26, 42, 50, 79, 87, 103, 109, 118

practical recommendations,
  behavioural neurology
  (all AEDs) 149t
pregabalin 7, 9t, 18, 93–9
  adverse effects 95, 96–7t
  behavioural/cognitive effects in
    epilepsy 98
  chronology of clinical use 94f
  dose titration 95
  generic formulation 93
  indications 93–4
  interactions, with alcohol/food 97
  overall rating 99t
  plasma levels monitoring 95
  pregnancy; hepatic and renal
    impairment 97–8
  preparations and
    structure 93–4f
  psychiatric use 98
  recommendations from
    NICE 94
primidone 7, 8t, 11–12, 77–84
  adverse effects 81t
  behavioural/cognitive effects in
    epilepsy 83–4
  chronology of clinical use 78f
  dose titration 79
  generic formulation 77
  indications 77–8
  interactions
    with AEDs 80–1
    with alcohol/food 82
    with other drugs 82
  overall rating 84
  plasma levels monitoring 79
  pregnancy; hepatic and renal
    impairment 82–3
  preparations and
    structure 77–8f
  psychiatric use 83f, 84
psychiatric use, indications
    (all AEDs) 148t
  comparative chart, level of
    evidence 150f
  temporal relationship with
    seizures 3
psychosis, effects of AEDs 148–9t
pyrrolidone derivatives 7, 8t

R

rufinamide 7, 9t, 19, 135–46
  adverse effects 138–9t
  behavioural/cognitive effects in
    epilepsy 145
  dose titration 137
  generic formulation 137
  indications 137
  interactions
    with AEDs 141
    with alcohol/food 142
    with other drugs 141
  pregnancy; hepatic and renal
    impairment 143–4
  preparations and structure 135f
  psychiatric use 145

S

Sabril® see vigabatrin
skin reactions 26, 44, 72, 80, 81,
  88, 119, 132
Stevens-Johnson syndrome 28,
  29, 31, 65, 72, 80, 81, 88,
  111, 119, 132, 139
substance abuse, effects of
  AEDs 149t

T

taste disturbance 28, 96, 110
Tegretol® see carbamazepine
tiagabine 7, 8t, 16, 101–6
  behavioural/cognitive effects in
    epilepsy 105
  cautions, adverse effects 103t
  chronology of clinical
    use 102f
  dose titration 102
  generic formulation 101
  indications 101
  interactions
    with AEDs 104
    with alcohol/food 104
    with other drugs 104
  overall rating 106t
  plasma levels monitoring 102
  pregnancy; hepatic and renal
    impairment 104–5
  preparations and
    structure 101–2f
  psychiatric use 106t
  recommendations from
    NICE 101
Topamax® see topiramate
topiramate 7, 8t, 16, 107–14
  behavioural/cognitive effects in
    epilepsy 113
  cautions, adverse
    effects 109–11t
  chronology of clinical use 108f
  dose titration 109
  generic formulation 107
  indications 107–8
  interactions
    with AEDs 111
    with alcohol/food 112
  overall rating 106t, 114
  plasma levels monitoring 109
  pregnancy; hepatic and renal
    impairment 112
  preparations and
    structure 107–8f
  psychiatric use 113
  recommendations from
    NICE 108
Trileptal® see oxcarbazepine

V

valproate 7, 8t, 13, 115–22
  behavioural/cognitive effects in
    epilepsy 121–2

cautions, adverse
  effects 117–19t
dose titration 117
generic formulation 116
indications 116
interactions
  with AEDs 119
  with alcohol/food 120
  with other drugs 120
overall rating 122t
plasma levels monitoring 117
pregnancy; hepatic and renal
  impairment 120–1
preparations and
  structure 115–16f
psychiatric use 121
recommendations from
  NICE 117
vigabatrin 7, 8t, 14, 123–8
  behavioural/cognitive effects in
    epilepsy 127
  cautions, adverse
    effects 125–6t
  dose titration 124
  generic formulation 124
  indications 124
  interactions
    with AEDs 126, 133
    with alcohol/food 126
  overall rating 128t
  plasma levels monitoring 117
  pregnancy; hepatic and renal
    impairment 126–7
  preparations and
    structure 123f
  psychiatric use 127f, 128
  recommendations from
    NICE 124
Vimpat® see lacosamide

Z

Zarontin® see ethosuximide
Zebinix® see eslicarbazepine
Zonegran® see zonisamide
zonisamide 7, 9t, 18, 129–34
  behavioural/cognitive effects in
    epilepsy 133–4
  cautions, adverse
    effects 131–2t
  dose titration 130
  generic formulation 129
  indications 130
  interactions
    with AEDs 132
    with alcohol/food/other
      drugs 133
  overall rating 134t
  plasma levels monitoring 131
  pregnancy; hepatic and renal
    impairment 133–4
  preparations and
    structure 129–30f
  psychiatric use 134f
  recommendations from
    NICE 130

The manufacturer's authorised representative in the EU for product safety is
Oxford University Press España S.A. of el Parque Empresarial San Fernando de
Henares, Avenida de Castilla, 2 – 28830 Madrid (www.oup.es/en or product.
safety@oup.com). OUP España S.A. also acts as importer into Spain of products
made by the manufacturer.

www.ingramcontent.com/pod-product-compliance
Ingram Content Group UK Ltd.
Pitfield, Milton Keynes, MK11 3LW, UK
UKHW021303180426
11947UKWH00015B/982